OXFORD MEDICAL PUBLICATIONS

Emergencies in Trauma

Published and forthcoming titles in the Emergencies in ... series:

Emergencies in Anaesthesia, Second Edition
Edited by Keith Allman, Andrew McIndoe, and Iain H. Wilson

Emergencies in Cardiology, Second Edition
Edited by Saul G. Myerson, Robin P. Choudhury, and Andrew Mitchell

Emergencies in Clinical Surgery
Edited by Chris Callaghan, J. Andrew Bradley, and Christopher Watson

Emergencies in Critical Care
Edited by Martin Beed, Richard Sherman, and Ravi Mahajan

Emergencies in Nursing
Edited by Philip Downing

Emergencies in Obstetrics and Gynaecology
Edited by S. Arulkumaran

Emergencies in Oncology
Edited by Martin Scott-Brown, Roy A.J. Spence, and Patrick G. Johnston

Emergencies in Paediatrics and Neonatology
Edited by Stuart Crisp and Jo Rainbow

Emergencies in Palliative and Supportive Care
Edited by David Currow and Katherine Clark

Emergencies in Primary Care
Chantal Simon, Karen O'Reilly, John Buckmaster, and Robin Proctor

Emergencies in Psychiatry
Basant K. Puri and Ian H. Treasaden

Emergencies in Clinical Radiology
Edited by Richard Graham and Ferdia Gallagher

Emergencies in Respiratory Medicine
Edited by Robert Parker, Catherine Thomas, and Lesley Bennett

Emergencies in Trauma
Aneel Bhangu, Caroline Lee, and Keith Porter

Head, Neck and Dental Emergencies
Edited by Mike Perry

Medical Emergencies in Dentistry
Nigel Robb and Jason Leitch

Emergencies in Trauma

Aneel Bhangu

ST3 General Surgery,
West Midlands Deanery

Caroline Lee

Specialist Registrar in Emergency Medicine
West Midlands

Keith Porter

Professor of Clinical Traumatology,
Queen Elizabeth Hospital,
Birmingham

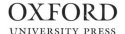

OXFORD
UNIVERSITY PRESS

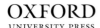

OXFORD
UNIVERSITY PRESS

Great Clarendon Street, Oxford OX2 6DP

Oxford University Press is a department of the University of Oxford.
It furthers the University's objective of excellence in research, scholarship,
and education by publishing worldwide in

Oxford New York

Auckland Cape Town Dar es Salaam Hong Kong Karachi
Kuala Lumpur Madrid Melbourne Mexico City Nairobi
New Delhi Shanghai Taipei Toronto

With offices in

Argentina Austria Brazil Chile Czech Republic France Greece
Guatemala Hungary Italy Japan Poland Portugal Singapore
South Korea Switzerland Thailand Turkey Ukraine Vietnam

Oxford is a registered trade mark of Oxford University Press
in the UK and in certain other countries

Published in the United States
by Oxford University Press Inc., New York

British Library Cataloguing in Publication Data
Data available

Library of Congress Cataloging in Publication Data
Data available

Typeset by Cepha Imaging Private Ltd., Bangalore, India
Printed in China
on acid-free paper through
Asia Pacific Offset

ISBN 978–0–19–955864–3

10 9 8 7 6 5 4 3 2 1

This book is dedicated to the trauma patient and to our colleagues who work tirelessly to save life and limb.

Foreword

Having been tasked by the Secretary of State for Health to construct health policy to implement the recommendations of the reports by the National Confidential Enquiry into Patient Outcome and Deaths, Trauma: who cares? (2007), this book is very welcome. It presents, in a most accessible format, the practical knowledge that will support those very critical early decisions which may ultimately determine the survival and outcome disability of patients with major trauma. It not only offers a valuable resource in the emergency assessment and care phase for junior doctors rotating through the emergency specialties, but it is also particularly useful in guiding assessment of specific orthopaedic emergencies and injuries. The book and chapter layout lends itself as a rapid reference document which is comprehensive, neatly referenced and of practical day-to-day use. I anticipate this will be one of those books with a well-worn cover by the end of any trauma clinical attachment.

We all recognise that we must move to consultant-led services for the reception and treatment of patients with serious injuries. However, this well-written text will foster well-prepared and briefed junior medical staff and present the opportunity to reflect on the care received in these often stressful emergency environments.

Professor Keith M Willett
Professor of Orthopaedic Trauma Surgery
Honorary Consultant Trauma and Orthopaedic Surgeon
Nuffield Department of Orthopaedic Surgery
University of Oxford

Preface

The ideas and principles of this book were born from the necessity to address two modern issues surrounding the management of trauma. Firstly, the skill-mix of junior doctors rotating through many departments has changed dramatically as a result of Modernising Medical Careers. Many orthopaedic and surgical specialities who manage trauma on a day-to-day basis now routinely have FY2 doctors and GP trainees passing through as part of modern rotations: posts which were previously filled by senior surgical SHOs. This is further exacerbated by Hospital at Night policies, where medical specialities may cover surgical patients. Secondly, the NCE-POD report "Trauma: who cares?" has identified shortfalls in the modern management of trauma within the United Kingdom, where there is still a need to reduce morbidity and mortality.

This book is essentially split into two halves. The first half deals with the management of general trauma topics, which are primarily the life-threatening issues. These are dealt with using a didactic, systematic approach, including which procedures to perform to preserve life and limb, and also when to contact senior help.

The second half of the book is dedicated to the recognition and management of the common fractures and emergency orthopaedic conditions which are encountered in day-to-day practice. We have avoided the two areas which bog down other such texts: complex classification systems and surgical technique. For example, when describing the initial management of fractures, we have only used classification systems where necessary for immediate management, and have listed surgical options rather than techniques. There are clear instructions on how to immobilise fractures, who can be sent home, and who needs to be admitted.

This book will help the junior doctor in the day-to-day management of all aspects of trauma. It will be beneficial for use in the Emergency Department, in Acute Assessment Areas, on the wards, and in Fracture Clinics. With clear information on how to recognize and manage sick trauma patients, how to initially manage fractures, and when to contact senior doctors, this text will be like 'having a consultant in your pocket.'

Contents

Abbreviations

ABCD	airway, breathing, circulation, disability
ABG	arterial blood gas
ACJ	acromioclavicular joint
ACL	anterior cruciate ligament
AF	atrial fibrillation
AFO	ankle-foot orthosis
AK	above knee
ALI	acute lung injury
ALS	advanced life support
AP	antero-posterior
APTT	activated partial thromboplastin time
ARDS	adult respiratory distress syndrome
ATLS	Advanced Trauma Life Support
AVN	avascular necrosis
AVPU	Alert, Voice, Pain, Unresponsive
bd	twice daily
B-E	below elbow
BK	below knee
BLS	basic life support
BM	Boehringer Mannheim test (a test for blood sugar levels)
BNF	British National Formulary
BP	blood pressure
BVM	bag valve mask
CK	creatinine kinase
CO	carbon monoxide
CO_2	carbon dioxide
COHb	carboxyhaemoglobin
COPD	chronic obstructive pulmonary disease
CPP	cerebral perfusion pressure
CPR	cardiopulmonary resuscitation
CRP	C-reactive protein
CSF	cerebrospinal fluid
CT	computed tomography (scan)
CTG	cardiotocography
CVA	cerebrovascular accident (stroke)
CVP	central venous pressure

CXR	chest X-ray
DDH	developmental dysplasia of the hip
DHS	dynamic hip screw
DIC	disseminated intravascular coagulopathy
DIPJ	distal interphalangeal joint
DPL	diagnostic peritoneal lavage
DRE	digital rectal examination
DVT	deep vein thrombosis
ECG	electrocardiogram
Echo	echocardiogram
ED	emergency department
ENT	ear nose and throat
EPB	extensor pollicis brevis
EPL	extensor pollicis longus
ESR	erythrocyte sedimentation rate
ETCO2	end tidal carbon dioxide
ETT	endotracheal tube
FAST	focused assessment with sonography for trauma
FBC	full blood count
FDP	flexor digitorum profundus
FDS	flexor digitorum superficialis
FFP	fresh frozen plasma
FOOSH	fall onto outstretched hand
FU	follow-up
FWB	fully weight bearing
G&S	group and save
GA	general anaesthetic
GCS	Glasgow coma score
GI	gastrointestinal
GP	general practitioner
GSW	gun shot wound
GT	greater tuberosity
H+	hydrogen ions
Hb	haemoglobin
HDU	high dependency unit
ICP	intracranial pressure
ICU	intensive care unit
IJ	internal jugular
IM	intramuscular
IO	intra-osseous

INR	International Normalized Ratio (of prothrombin time)
ITU	intensive treatment unit
IV	intravenous
IVC	Inferior vena cava
IVI	intravenous infusion
JVP	jugular venous pressure
LA	local anaesthetic
LFT	liver function tests
LMA	laryngeal mask airway
LOC	loss of consciousness
LMWH	low molecular weight heparin
MAP	mean arterial blood pressure
MCJP	metacarpophalangeal joints
MDU	Medical Defense Union
mg	milligrams
MI	myocardial infarction
MILS	manual in-line stabilisation
MIST	Mechanism, Injury, Symptoms and signs, Treatment
MPS	Medical Protection Society
MUA	manipulation under anaesthesia
NAI	non-accidental injury
NBM	nil by mouth
NCEPOD	National Confidential Enquiry into Patient Outcome and Death
NG	nasogastric
NGT	nasogastric tube
NIBP	non-invasive blood pressure
NPA	nasopharyngeal airway
NSAID	non-steroidal anti-inflammatory drug
NWB	non-weight bearing
O_2	oxygen
O&G	obstetrics and gynaecology
OCP	oral contraceptive pill
od	once daily
OPA	oropharyngeal airway
ORIF	open reduction, internal fixation
$PaCO_2$	partial pressure of carbon dioxide in arterial blood
PaO_2	partial pressure of oxygen in arterial blood
pCO_2	partial pressure of carbon dioxide
PE	pulmonary embolus
PEA	pulseless electrical activity

PIPJ	proximal interphalangeal joint
PMH	past medical history
po	by mouth
pO_2	partial pressure of oxygen
PoP	plaster of Paris
PPI	proton pump inhibitor
PR	per rectum
prn	as needed
PV	per vaginam
PWB	partial weight bearing
qds	four times a day
RBBB	right bundle branch block
RBC	red blood cells
RSI	rapid sequence induction
RTC	road traffic collision
SaO_2	O_2 arterial saturation
SBP	systolic blood pressure
sc	subcutaneous
SC	subclavian
SI	sacro-iliac
SOB	short of breath
SpR	specialist registrar
ST	specialist trainee
SUFE	slip of the femoral epiphysis
SCIWORA	spinal cord injury without radiological abnormality
T&O	trauma and orthopaedics
TBSA	total body surface area
tds	three times a day
TEDS	thrombo-embolic deterrent stockings
TOE	transoesophageal echocardiogram
TTE	transthoracic echocardiogram
U&E	urea and electrolytes
USS	ultrasound scan
VF	ventricular fibrillation
WB	weight bearing
WBC	white blood cells
WCC	white cell count
X-match	cross-match blood

Normal values

Note that 'normal' values in adults may vary slightly between laboratories. Normal values in pregnancy are shown on page 110.

Arterial blood gas analysis

pH	7.35–7.45
pO_2	>10.6 kPa, 75–100 mmHg
pCO_2	4.5–6.0 kPa, 35–45 mmHg
bicarbonate	24–28 mmol/L
base excess	±2 mmol/L

Biochemistry

alanine aminotransferase (ALT)	5–35 IU/L
albumin	35–50 g/L
alanine phosphatase	30–300 IU/L
amylase	0–180 U/dL
aspartate transaminase (AST)	5–35 IU/L
bicarbonate	24–30 mmol/L
bilirubin	3–17 µmol/L
calcium (total)	2.12–2.65 mmol/L
calcium (ionized)	1–1.25 mmol/L
chloride	95–105 mmol/L
creatine kinase (CK)	25–195 IU/L
creatinine	70–150 µmol/L
C-reactive protein (CRP)	<3 mg/L
glucose (fasting)	35–5.5 mmol/L
magnesium	0.75–1.05 mmol/L
osmolality	278–305 mosmol/kg
potassium	3.5–5.0 mmol/L
sodium	135–145 mmol/L
urea	2.5–6.7 mmol/L
urate (female)	150–390 µmol/L
urate (male)	210–480 µmol/L

Haematology

Hb (women)	11.5–16.0 g/dL
Hb (men)	13.5–18.0 g/dL
Hct (women)	0.37–0.47
Hct (men)	0.40–0.54
MCV	76 96 femtol
WCC	$4.0–11.0 \times 10^9$/L
neutrophils	$2.0–7.5 \times 10^9$/L (40–75% of WCC)
lymphocytes	$1.5–4.0 \times 10^9$/L (20–40% of WCC)
monocytes	$0.2–0.8 \times 10^9$/L (2–10% of WCC)
eosinophils	$0.04–0.40 \times 10^9$/L (1–6% of WCC)
basophils	$<0.1 \times 10^9$/L (<1% of WCC)

Haematology-continued

platelets	$150–400 \times 10^9/L$
prothrombin time	12–15 s
(factors I, II, VII, X)	
APTT (factors VII, IX, XI, XII)	23–42 s

International Normalized Ratio (INR)

2.0–3.0	for treating DVT, pulmonary embolism
2.5–3.5	embolism prophylaxis for AF
3.0–4.0	recurrent thromboembolic disease, arterial grafts and prosthetic valves
ESR (women)	<(age in years + 10)/2 mm/h
ESR (men)	<(age in years)/2 mm/h

Metric conversion

Length

1 m = 3 feet 3.4 inches	1 foot = 0.3048 m
1 cm = 0.394 inch	1inch = 25.4 mm

Weight

1 kg = 2.20 lb	1 stone = 6.35 kg
1 g = 15.4 grains	1 lb = 0.454 kg

Volume

1 L = 1.76 UK pints = 2.11 US liquid pints
1 UK pints = 20 fl oz = 0.568 L
1 US liquid pint = 16 fl oz = 0.473 L
1 teaspoon = 5 mL
1 tablespoon = 15 mL

Temperature

Temperature in °C = (temperature in °F − 32) × 5/9
Pressure 1 kPa = 7.5 mmHg

Paediatric values

Age (years)	Pulse	Respiratory rate
<1	110–160	30–40
2–5	95–140	25–30
5–12	80–120	20–25
>12	60–100	15–20

Part 1

Trauma

Principles of trauma management

⑦ The Trauma team

The members of the hospital Trauma team will vary between individual trusts depending on the resources and personnel available and the time of day. The NCEPOD Report 'Trauma: who cares?' published in 2007 recommended that a Trauma team should be available 24 h a day, 7 days a week, and a consultant must be the team leader for the management of the severely-injured patient.

Preparing for the patient

Alert and assemble team

- Send out trauma alert to on-call members of Trauma team via switchboard.
- Trauma team leader allocates predetermined roles on arrival.

Personal protective equipment

All hands-on staff should be wearing gloves, apron, eye protection/facemasks, and a lead apron for primary survey X-rays.

Prepare monitoring and medical equipment

- Prepare 3 lead echocardiogram (ECG), and monitor blood pressure (BP) and O_2 arterial saturation (SaO_2).
- Collect equipment for wide bore intravenous access and phlebotomy.
- Run 2 L of warmed sodium chloride 0.9% fluid through large giving sets ready to administer if required.
- Ensure the portable emergency ultrasound machine is available in the Resuscitation room if there is one in your department.

Alert other departments

- Radiographer for chest and pelvis X-ray in the Resuscitation room.
- Computed tomography (CT) radiographer/radiologist.
- Blood bank.
- Theatres.

Roles in the team

Trauma team leader

- Leads resuscitation.
- Decides on patient management.
- Prioritizes investigations and treatment.
- Liaises with specialists.
- Normally consultant or minimum SpR level.

Anaesthetist

- Assessment and management of airway.
- Administers oxygen and ventilation.
- Responsible for cervical spine immobilization and control of log roll.
- Takes **ample** history in alert patients. 📖 AMPLE history, p70.

Nurse 1
- Applies monitoring equipment including ECG leads, SaO$_2$ probe, BP cuff.
- Assists with procedures.

Nurse 2
- Removes clothes from patient starting with chest and upper limbs.
- Assists with procedures.

Doctor 1
- Conducts primary survey from B-E and informs Trauma team leader.
- Performs procedures depending on skill and training.

Doctor 2
- Obtains IV access and sends off bloods.
- Performs procedures depending on skill and training.

Scribe
Documents history and all clinical findings.

Specialists
Includes senior general surgeon, senior orthopaedic surgeon, and other specialists to provide expert opinions as required.

Arrival of the patient
Allow the ambulance crew to give a rapid handover to all members of the Trauma team before transferring the patient, and starting assessment or interventions. The exception to this rule are patients requiring immediate airway management or ongoing cardiopulmonary resuscitation (CPR).

The ambulance service handover will usually follow the MIST format and should take no more than 20 s:
- Mechanism of injury.
- Injuries suspected or found.
- Signs and symptoms.
- Treatment given.

⑦ The primary survey

The primary survey is a rapid structured assessment designed to identify and treat any injuries that could be immediately life-threatening. Resuscitation is performed simultaneously as problems are identified.

The primary survey follows the ABCDE format:

A airway with cervical spine control
B breathing with ventilation and oxygen
C circulation and haemorrhage control
D disability
E exposure

NB. In the presence of catastrophic external haemorrhage C takes priority over A and B. The doctor should return to the ABC after control of this haemorrhage, e.g. application of a tourniquet for limb exsanguination.

Airway with cervical spine control

- Talk to the patient and assess their response. Listen for any noisy breathing to suggest an obstructed airway. Look inside the mouth and use suction to remove any foreign bodies or debris.
- Avoid tilting the head if there is any chance of a cervical spine injury.
- Provide manual in-line stabilization using a hand on either side of the patient's head to hold the neck in a neutral position, or use a cervical collar, blocks, and tape to immobilize the cervical spine.
- Use a jaw thrust or basic adjuncts [nasopharyngeal airway (NPA), oropharyngeal airway (OPA)] to open the airway. Call for senior Emergency department or anaesthetic support if the airway is compromised.

Breathing with ventilation and oxygen

- Give all major trauma patients 15 L O_2 via a mask with a non-rebreath reservoir bag.
- Count the respiratory rate.
- Expose the chest, and inspect for any deformity, wounds, asymmetrical chest movement, flail segments, or bruising.
- Palpate the chest along the clavicles, sternum, and ribs to assess for any tenderness, crepitus, or subcutaneous emphysema.
- Percuss the chest to detect hyper-resonance or dullness.
- Auscultate the chest with the patient taking an inspiratory effort or the anaesthetist ventilating the patient to assess the presence of breath sounds bilaterally.
- Ventilate patients using a bag-valve-mask if self-ventilation is inadequate.
- Decompress tension pneumothoraces with needle thoracocentesis and cover open pneumothoraces.

Circulation with haemorrhage control

- Assess radial pulse, pulse rate, and BP.
- Identify and control any external bleeding.
- Inspect the abdomen for any pattern bruising or distension, and palpate for tenderness.
- Inspect the pelvis for any bruising, deformity, or swelling, and any perineal wounds or genital bleeding.
- Inspect and palpate both femurs for deformity, swelling, tenderness, or wounds.
- Establish 2 × IV access and send bloods including full blood count (FBC), urea and electrolytes (U&E), liver function tests (LFT), amylase, clotting, and X-match.
- Commence IV fluids if patient is hypotensive.

Disability

- Assess Glasgow Coma Score (GCS) and pupils.
- Check BM and temperature.
- Safely logroll the patient off the spinal board if appropriate. Check the back for any wounds, and palpate down the thoracic and lumbar spine for any tenderness in a conscious patient. Check anal tone and sensation if any suspicion of spinal injury.
- **NB.** Logroll should be avoided in hypotensive trauma patients, those with suspected intrathoracic or abdominal bleeding, or those with probable pelvic fractures to avoid clot disruption and further haemorrhage. Transfer with a scoop stretcher or PAT slide is safer.

Exposure

- Undress the patient to allow full examination and identification of any other injuries.
- Keep warm.
- Give analgesia.
- Cover wounds, apply splints.

Following an initial rapid primary survey, the patient may undergo primary investigations or be moved straight to theatre for resuscitative surgery.

⊘ Adjuncts to the primary survey

Investigations in the primary survey should strictly be limited to those where the results will change the immediate management of the patient.

Chest X-ray

A supine chest X-ray (CXR) will identify any large pneumothorax, haemothorax causing hypovolaemic shock, or mediastinal enlargement.

Pelvic X-ray

A pelvic X-ray will identify any significant fractures causing hypovolaemic shock, which can be managed early with splintage.

It is often useful to ask the radiographer to pre-load the trolley with films prior to the arrival of the patient.

Emergency ultrasound

A trained operator can perform a focused assessment with sonography for trauma (FAST) scan during the primary survey. This includes detection of free fluid in the abdomen (between the right kidney and liver, between the left kidney and spleen, and in the pelvis) and detection of pericardial fluid around the heart.

The FAST scan is mostly useful for haemodynamically unstable patients in determining an indication for emergency laparotomy or thoracotomy. It may be falsely negative if performed early as sufficient intra-abdominal blood may not have collected in dependent areas, and is operator dependent. Ultrasound can also be used to detect the presence of pleural fluid or pneumothorax.

Emergency ultrasound has superseded diagnostic peritoneal lavage for the detection of intra-abdominal bleeding in the developed world.

Arterial blood gases

Blood gases are important to identify the adequacy of oxygenation and ventilation and may guide the need for intubation and invasive ventilation. They also provide useful information about the degree of acidosis and some machines may give a rapid measurement of haemoglobin (Hb).

Echocardiogram

Medical conditions, e.g. myocardial infarction (MI), arrhythmia, occasionally present as the cause of a RTC or fall from height, and need to be excluded. Chest injuries may cause cardiac contusions. Acidosis from hypovolaemia may cause arrhythmias. Older patients >50 years should routinely have an ECG performed to identify pre-existing medical conditions.

Urinalysis

Most major trauma patients will require catheterization to monitor hourly urine outputs and fluid balance. Ensure the patient does not have a pelvic fracture or urethral injury before attempting catheterization.

Dipstick of the urine may reveal microscopic haematuria, which may indicate an intra-abdominal injury.

A urine pregnancy test should be performed on all females of child-bearing age.

Computed tomography

CT is a valuable resource, which can be used to detect occult life-threatening injuries. It is also useful to detect solid-organ injuries, which can be treated conservatively, or to diagnose vascular injuries for surgery or interventional radiology. Modern multi-slice spiral CT scanners are now able to perform scans of the head, neck, chest, abdomen, and pelvis in a matter of minutes.

Many trauma centres now advocate 'whole body CT' for patients according to a protocol depending on the mechanism of injury. This has raised some concerns regarding radiation doses for the patient and long-term sequelae.

The Trauma team should accompany the patient to the CT scanner when used in the primary survey.

Haemodynamically unstable patients should only be taken to CT under the care of a senior experienced surgeon, accompanied by cross-matched blood and in the vicinity of an immediately available theatre.

⑦ **Secondary survey**

The secondary survey is a systematic head to toe examination to identify any other injuries. It should only be performed after the primary survey has been completed, all life-threatening injuries have been excluded, and the patient is stable. For this reason, some patients do not have a secondary survey performed until the post-operative period.

AMPLE history

- Allergies.
- Medication.
- Past medical history.
- Last ate or drank.
- Events leading up to injury – what do they remember?

Head and maxillofacial

- Check the scalp and head for any wounds, bruising, or swelling.
- Revaluate GCS.
- Assess the eyes for foreign bodies (including contact lenses, which need removal), visual acuity, pupil size and reactivity, conjunctival haemorrhage or hyphaema, penetrating injury, range of movements of the eye. If there is facial oedema, the eyelids will need to be prised open to exclude any ocular injury.
- Assess the nose and ears for haemorrhage or cerebrospinal fluid (CSF) leakage.
- Assess cranial nerve function.
- Palpate over the face for any bony tenderness.
- Assess the mouth for evidence of bleeding, intra-oral lacerations, or dental injury.

Cervical spine and neck

- Inspect and palpate the neck for tracheal deviation, wounds, subcutaneous emphysema, laryngeal crepitus, or distended neck veins.
- Palpate and ausculate over the carotid artery.
- With manual in-line stabilization performed by an assistant, palpate the posterior cervical vertebrae for tenderness. **NB.** The cervical spine cannot be cleared clinically in the presence of other distracting injuries or a reduced conscious level (see 📖 Cervical spine injury, p22).

Chest

- Inspect, palpate, percuss, and auscultate the chest again. Check the front, back, and sides, including the axillary regions.
- Assess heart sounds and jugular venous pressure (JVP).
- Recheck the CXR performed in the primary survey.

Abdomen

- Inspect the anterior abdomen and posterior flanks.
- Palpate the abdomen for tenderness.
- Listen for bowel sounds.
- Inspect the perineum and genitals for bruising or bleeding. Perform an internal rectal (and in selected cases vaginal) examination with a chaperone if there is any suspicion of abdominal, pelvic, or spinal cord injury.

Musculoskeletal

- Inspect, palpate, and move all four limbs to identify swelling, tenderness or abnormal movements from injury.
- Check peripheral pulses.
- Reassess the pelvis after reviewing the pelvic X-ray from the primary survey.
- Inspect and palpate the thoracic and lumbar spine for tenderness.
- Obtain X-rays for any suspected limb or spinal fractures not already imaged.

Neurological status

- Evaluate the power, tone and sensation of all four limbs.
- Assess anal tone and sensation in patients with suspected spinal injury if not already performed.

Specialized diagnostic tests may be required following the secondary survey to identify specific injuries, e.g. X-rays, CT, or contrast urography or arteriography. Make sure all your findings are clearly documented on the trauma chart or patients medical records.

Tertiary survey

There is a high rate of missed injuries in trauma patients, especially those who are unconscious or haemodynamically unstable or who have distracting major injuries. It is therefore recommended that a systematic head to toe reassessment is performed on ICU or on the ward, within 24 h of the patient's admission.

Airway

☠ **Airway management**

Airway obstruction is a common finding in trauma patients and may lead to early preventable deaths. The airway is the first priority in resuscitation. As well as identifying actual airway obstruction it is important to identify a potential for deterioration and to obtain senior anaesthetic support early.

Causes of airway obstruction in trauma
- Reduced conscious level (tongue).
- Foreign body.
- Vomit or blood.
- Facial injury.
- Laryngeal fracture.
- Burns.

Assessment
- **Look** inside the mouth for oedema, burns, foreign bodies, fluids, or bleeding. Inspect the face and neck for burns, swelling, or wounds. Look at the patient generally for signs of agitation or a reduced conscious level. Use of accessory muscles, tracheal tug, or see-sawing abdominal breathing may also indicate airway obstruction.
- **Listen** to breath sounds at the mouth for snoring (soft tissue obstruction), gurgling (fluids), stridor, or a hoarse voice.
- **Feel** the facial bones for fractures, and the neck for swelling, emphysema or palpable laryngeal fractures.

Basic airway management
- If the patient is talking to you with a normal voice, no immediate management is required.
- If the patient is obtunded, open the mouth and inspect.
- Suction any fluids, or remove solids with Magill's forceps.
- If patient vomits, call for help and perform rapid log roll onto side to clear airway.

If the patient has an obstructed airway, perform a jaw thrust by lifting the angles of the lower jaw forward (Fig. 2.1). Do not use a head tilt – chin lift manoeuvre in trauma patients with a risk of cervical spine injury. If obstruction persists use an airway adjunct. The options are an oropharyngeal airway (OPA) or nasopharyngeal airway (NPA).

Oropharyngeal airway (Fig. 2.2a)
- Useful in an unconscious patient with no gag reflex.
- Size length by measuring distance from centre of incisors to angle of jaw. Insert upside down and rotate 180° to lie over the tongue.
- In children insert concave down with direct vision using a tongue depressor to avoid damage to soft tissues.
- If insertion provokes any gagging or coughing the OPA must be removed immediately to prevent vomiting and aspiration.

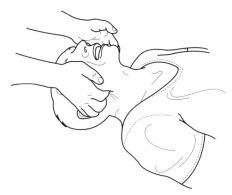

Fig. 2.1 Jaw thrust.

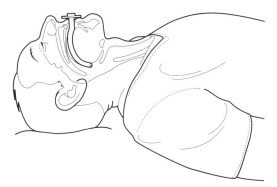

Fig. 2.2 (a) Oropharyngeal airway.

Nasopharyngeal airway (Fig. 2.2b)

- Often better tolerated by semi-conscious patients and especially useful for patients who have trismus following a head injury.
- Size 6 in average female and size 7 in average male.
- Ideally insert in right nostril, but aim for the largest unobstructed nostril. Lubricate and insert perpendicular to the face with a gentle rotatory motion.
- Do not force the NPA in against any obstruction or bleeding will occur from the nasal mucosa, which may further compromise the airway. Try the other nostril or a smaller size if any resistance occurs.
- Use caution in patients with suspected basal skull fracture or maxillary fractures.

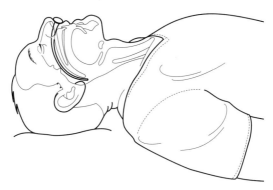

Fig. 2.2 (b) Nasopharyngeal airway.

Laryngeal mask airway

The laryngeal mask airway (LMA) is a tube with a spoon-shaped inflatable cuff at the distal end, which can be inserted blindly into the airway. The tip of the cuff sits in the entrance to the oesophagus and channels air into the laryngeal inlet. The LMA is sized according to the estimated weight of the patient.

It is used as a temporary measure to maintain an airway in an unconscious patient who requires tracheal intubation or as a failed intubation device to allow re-oxygenation.

The device requires training before use to ensure correct placement. It is not appropriate in patients with a gag reflex or vomiting, and will not ventilate the patient effectively if they require high pressures.

☠ The definitive airway

A definitive airway is defined as 'a cuffed tube inflated in the trachea'. Orotracheal intubation is the gold standard for providing a definitive airway.

The majority of patients will require rapid sequence intubation facilitated by anaesthetic drugs. This should only be attempted by physicians who are appropriately trained and experienced. It is better for the junior physician to use effective basic airway management skills to maintain a patent airway and wait for the arrival of a senior airway specialist. Patients who can be intubated without drugs are unlikely to survive.

Indications for tracheal intubation

- Reduced conscious level.
- Obstructed airway.
- Prevent potential obstruction (e.g. from burns or airway injury).
- Risk of aspiration.
- Apnoea.
- Inadequate oxygenation or ventilation, e.g. chest injury.

Assisting with RSI

Preparation
- **Equipment**: prepare and check all equipment for oxygen delivery (BVM), suction, routine intubation (endotracheal tube, working laryngoscope, 10-mL syringe, tie) difficult intubation (bougie, McCoys larygnoscope), and failed intubation (LMA, surgical airway kit).
- **Monitoring**: continuous ECG, pulse oximetry, non-invasive blood pressure (NIBP), end tidal CO_2 ($ETCO_2$).
- Assess patients AMPLE history, ensure 2× IV access working, and check neurological status, e.g. GCS, pupils, and moving all four limbs prior to paralysis.
- **Patient positioning**: trauma patients require continuous cervical spine immobilization. During the rapid sequence induction (RSI), the collar is removed and manual in-line stabilization performed by an assistant who crouches to the side of the patient.
- **Briefing** of team members by the person leading the RSI to assign roles including intubation, drug administration, and watching monitors, cricoid pressure, and manual in-line stabilization (MILS). Explain the plan for failed intubation.

Pre-oxygenation
Ideally for at least three minutes to maximize the time before desaturation occurs when the patient becomes apnoeic.

Application of cricoid pressure
Maintained until the intubating physician has verbally confirmed correct tube placement.

Drug administration
An induction agent to produce loss of consciousness, followed by a rapid-acting neuromuscular blocking drug to produce paralysis. The doses of these are usually at least halved in patients with hypovolaemic shock.

Intubation
A maximum of 30 s for attempt or until patient desaturates below 92% before bag valve mask (BVM) ventilation is recommenced.

Confirmation of tube position
• The gold standard is $ETCO_2$ monitoring.
• Other checks are visual confirmation of the tube passing through the vocal cords, symmetrical chest movement, and good breath sounds bilaterally.
• Once tracheal intubation is confirmed and the cuff is inflated, the cricoid pressure can be released and the tube tied in position. Tape is often preferred to a ribbon tie, which can obstruct venous return in the neck if tied firmly.

Post-intubation
• Reassess vital signs.
• Request a CXR to check the position of the tube. Maintain anaesthesia by an infusion.
• Check ABG and consider an arterial line to provide continuous invasive BP measurements and a port for regular blood sampling.

Complications of intubation
• Hypotension from induction agents.
• Unsuccessful intubation with inability to ventilate patient.
• Intubation of right main bronchus if tube inserted too far.
• Tension pneumothorax if positive pressure ventilation delivered in the presence of an occult pneumothorax.
• Raised intracranial pressure in patients with head injury if inadequate drugs.

☢ Needle and surgical cricothyroidotomy

Indication
Complete upper airway obstruction or failed intubation with severe hypoxia, and inability to oxygenate or ventilate the patient via any other method.

Needle cricothyroidotomy
This is only a temporary life-saving measure as the narrow bore of the cannula will only partially oxygenate the patient and not provide any ventilation leading to CO_2 retention. It should be replaced as soon as possible by a surgical airway or intubation by an experienced practitioner.

Equipment
- 14G intravenous cannula.
- 10-mL syringe.
- Delivery system (a length of green oxygen tubing attached to a 2-mL syringe which can be connected to the venflon, a hole cut in the tubing just below the syringe, which can be occluded by a finger, and the other end attached to an oxygen supply)

Procedure
- Locate the cricothyroid membrane (see Fig. 2.3), and stabilize the larynx with the thumb and index finger of the non-dominant hand. Rapidly clean the skin with an alcohol wipe if available.
- Using the cannula attached to the syringe, puncture the skin in the midline over the cricothyroid membrane, aspirating as the needle is advanced at 45° pointing inferiorly.
- When air is freely aspirated, advance the cannula over the needle into the trachea and remove the needle.
- Aspirate again with the syringe to confirm the cannula is still in the trachea.
- Attach the delivery system to the venflon and occlude the hole for 1 s followed by 4 s off.
- Call an anaesthetist and senior ENT doctor and prepare equipment for surgical cricothyroidotomy.

Surgical cricothyroidotomy
This procedure allows insertion of a definitive airway. It should not be performed in pre-pubertal children as the cricoid cartilage is the only circumferential support to the upper trachea.

Equipment
Scalpel, Spencer Wells forceps, or tracheal dilators, size 6 cuffed tracheostomy tube (or use endotracheal tube with bougie), 10-mL syringe, BVM, stethoscope, tape.

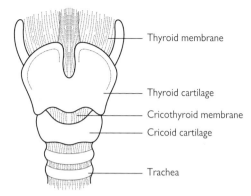

Fig. 2.3 Anatomy of the cricothyroid membrane.

Procedure
- Locate the cricothyroid membrane in the midline, and stabilize the larynx with thumb and index finger of non-dominant hand.
- Make a transverse incision in the skin and through the cricothyroid membrane using a scalpel. **Do not lose the hole!**
- Use Spencer Wells forceps or tracheal dilator to enlarge the hole.
- Insert a size 6 tracheostomy tube into the trachea.
- If this is not available pass a bougie into the trachea and railroad a 6-mm cuffed endotracheal tube over the bougie.
- Inflate the cuff and ventilate to check tube position as for orotracheal intubation.
- Secure the tube securely with tape.

Complications
- Failed insertion with hypoxia.
- Haemorrhage into airway with aspiration or soft tissues creating haematoma.
- Surgical emphysema.
- Posterior tracheal wall perforation.
- Oesophageal perforation.
- Air trapping with needle cricothyroidotomy (inadequate exhalation causes reduced venous return and hypotension).
- Late complications include infection, subglottic stenosis, and vocal cord paralysis.

☠ Cervical spine injury

Mechanism of injury
- High energy road traffic collision (RTC).
- Fall greater than 1½ times the patients vertical height.
- Diving into shallow water.
- Fall from a horse or collapse of a rugby scrum.
- Fall from a standing height in the elderly.

The possibility of cervical spine injury should be considered in every trauma patient. Early immobilization may prevent a potential spinal cord injury from occurring.

Spinal immobilization should be provided in:
- Every major blunt trauma patient.
- Penetrating trauma patients who have also sustained blunt trauma, e.g. fall from height to escape assailant.
- Patients with head injury and reduced conscious level.
- Minor trauma patients with midline neck tenderness or neurology, or who have pre-existing neck pathology.

In addition, have a low threshold for immobilization of elderly patients or intoxicated patients where the history of injury is not clear.

Evaluation of the cervical spine only takes place after life-threatening ABCD conditions have been excluded or managed.

Cervical spine immobilization
- The majority of trauma patients will arrive in the department immobilized by ambulance service personnel in a collar, head blocks, and straps, on a spinal board with body straps.
- If there are none in place, apply MILS with a gloved hand on either side of the head in a neutral position; avoid the ears to allow communication with the patient. Request a collar, head board, head blocks, and straps to immobilize the patient supine on the trolley if it is indicated.
- Agitated unco-operative patients should not have their cervical spine immobilized alone as greater injury can result from movements of the body on a restricted head.
- Remove patients from a spinal board as soon as possible (after the primary survey) to avoid development of pressure sores and improve the patient's comfort.

Log-rolling

Patients with no suspicion of internal bleeding (chest, abdomen, pelvis, femurs), who have stable vital signs can be log-rolled at the end of the primary survey.

This allows assessment of the spine and posterior torso for injury, and removal off the long board. One person is responsible for holding the head in MILS and co-ordinating the log roll as team leader. Three people hold (1) the patients shoulders and waist, (2) the patients hips and under the uppermost thigh, and (3) both hands under the uppermost leg. The roll to 45° is performed on the team leaders instructions. The fifth person pulls out the board, clears debris from under the patient, examines the back, palpates down the vertebral column for tenderness, and assesses anal tone and sensation where indicated. When completed the log roll team leader will give instructions and the patient is returned to a supine position.

Clearing the cervical spine

Major trauma patients

If the patient has multiple injuries and a CT scan is being performed, the cervical spine is usually imaged as part of the trauma series.

Minor trauma

Only consider clearing the neck when the primary survey is normal and the following criteria are met:

- Low risk mechanism of injury, e.g. low speed rear end shunt.
- No distracting injury.
- GCS 15, alert and orientated, with no drug or alcohol intoxication.
- No neurology in limbs (power, tone, sensation, and reflexes).
- No midline tenderness.
- No history of previous neck fracture or inflammatory joint disease, e.g. rheumatoid arthritis affecting neck.
- If none of the above, can rotate neck actively 45° left and right without pain.

If any of these criteria are positive the patient requires plain X-rays of the cervical spine in three views: antero-posterior (AP), open mouth odontoid peg view, and lateral X-ray from the base of the occiput to the top of T1 vertebrae.

If plain films are inadequate, abnormal, or there is still clinical suspicion despite a normal X-ray, a CT cervical spine should be requested.

☠ **Management of cervical spine injury**

Airway with cervical spine control

- Airways may be compromised due to direct trauma or decreased consciousness due to head injury. Even if the patient was brought in without spinal control immobilization – **immobilize if in doubt.**
- Consider intubation for those patients with a GCS of 8 or less (undertaken with the collar off and MILS) or combative head injury patients, to secure the airway, facilitate assessment, and protect the spine.

Breathing

- **Remember to assess for other chest injuries**.
- The phrenic nerve originates from C3 to C5, so respiratory failure is imminent if the patient is paralysed. Mechanical ventilation may be needed. Even with lower cervical spine injuries (e.g. C6), ascending oedema within the spinal cord may affect the phrenic segments.
- Patients with upper thoracic cord injuries and loss of intercostal function may suffer respiratory compromise.

Circulation

- Patients with spinal cord injuries (usually above T6) may suffer neurogenic shock. This occurs due to a loss of sympathetic tone and presents as hypotension, bradycardia, and warm dilated peripheries below the level of the cord.
- This does not exclude other injuries producing hypovolaemia (e.g. splenic injuries).

Disability

- Document and reassess GCS in patients with major trauma.
- Log roll in the secondary survey and assess for wounds, swelling, mid-line tenderness, vertebral steps, and mal-aligned spinous processes.
- Assess neurology fully. Consider upper and lower limb tone, power, reflexes, sensation, and co-ordination.
- PR to assess anal tone and to determine peri-anal sensation. Note faecal incontinence and lax sphincters.

Initial management

- IV access and titrated opiate analgesia if required.
- Catheterize to protect the bladder and monitor urine output.
- Image the spine. Be familiar with local protocols. Major trauma patients (especially those who are intubated) may require a CT of the whole spine as part of the trauma series. **Remember, with a single spinal fracture there is a 15% incidence of a second non-contiguous bony injury.**
- Consult regional spinal trauma units early for advice.
- Ileus is common and a nasogastric tube may be needed.

Common muscle groups and movements

- **C5:** elbow flexion (biceps) and shoulder abduction (deltoid).
- **C6:** wrist extension.
- **C7:** elbow extension (triceps).
- **C8:** middle finger flexion.
- **T1:** small finger abduction.
- **L2:** hip extension.
- **L3:** knee extension.
- **L4:** ankle dorsiflexion.
- **L5:** big toe extension.
- **S1:** ankle plantar flexion.

Common reflex arcs

- **C5/6:** biceps jerk.
- **C7/8:** triceps jerk.
- **C5/6:** supinator.
- **L3/4:** knee jerk.
- **S1/2:** ankle jerk.

Dermatomes (Fig. 2.4)

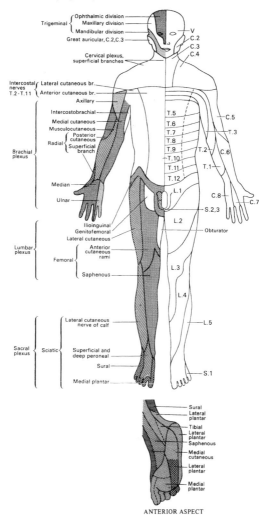

Fig. 2.4 Dermatomes. Reproduced from Longmore M et al. *Oxford Handbook of Clinical Medicine*, 7th Edition, 2007, with permission from Oxford University Press.

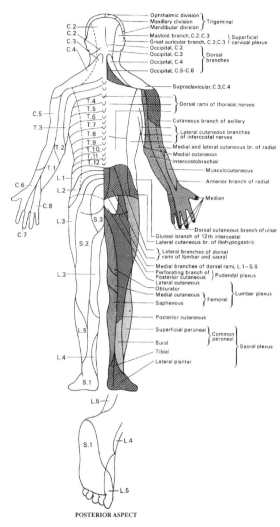

Ophthalmic division ⎫
Maxillary division ⎬ Trigeminal
Mandibular division ⎭
Mastoid branch, C.2, C.3 ⎫ Superficial
Great auricular branch, C.2, C.3 ⎬ cervical plexus
Occipital, C.2 ⎫
Occipital, C.3 ⎬ Dorsal
Occipital, C.4 ⎭ branches
Occipital, C.5–C.8

Supraclavicular, C.3, C.4

Dorsal rami of thoracic nerves

Cutaneous branch of axillary

Lateral cutaneous branches ⎫
of intercostal nerves ⎭

Medial and lateral cutaneous br. of radial
Medial cutaneous
Intercostobrachial

Musculocutaneous

Anterior branch of radial

Median

Dorsal cutaneous branch of ulnar
Gluteal branch of 12th intercostal
Lateral cutaneous br. of iliohypogastric
Lateral branches of dorsal ⎫
rami of lumbar and sacral ⎭
Medial branches of dorsal rami, L.1–S.6
Perforating branch of ⎫ Pudendal plexus
Posterior cutaneous ⎭
Lateral cutaneous
Obturator ⎫
Medial cutaneous ⎬ Femoral ⎫ Lumbar plexus
Saphenous ⎭

Posterior cutaneous

Superficial peroneal ⎫ Common
⎭ peroneal ⎫ Sacral plexus
Sural
Tibial
Lateral plantar

POSTERIOR ASPECT

Fig. 2.4 Cont'd

⑦ Interpreting X-rays of the spine

Interpreting spinal X-rays can be difficult and requires a system for reliable interpretation. Subsequent clinical management is focused around the stability of the injury – unstable fractures require initial immobilization with subsequent fixation in some cases, while stable fractures can be treated conservatively, often with early mobilization. The radiological findings must be correlated with the clinical picture.

Cervical spine

There are three films in the classical trauma series: lateral, AP, and open mouth view. The lateral is the most useful and widely used, the AP film adds information to the lateral, and the open mouth view shows the odontoid peg.

The ABCs method for interpreting lateral C-spine X-rays

- Adequacy and alignment: an adequate film shows C1–C7/T1 junction. If C7/T1 can't be seen, try pulling down the shoulders or obtain swimmer's views. Look for alignment of the vertebral contours to form 4 lines (Fig. 2.5). Disruption to these lines may indicate fracture or dislocation. Steps >25% of the vertebral body's width indicate unifacet dislocation; >50% indicates bifacet dislocation.
- **Bones:** trace all the bones for disruptions indicating fractures. Look at density for abnormalities, including crush injuries.
- **Cartilages:** look at the intervertebral discs to ensure they are of a uniform height. The space between the peg and lateral masses of C1 should be 3–5 mm and symmetrical.
- **Soft tissues:** look at the soft tissues for swellings and bony fragments. In front of C2, there should be 3 mm of soft tissue and in front of C6, 2 cm is the maximum width of soft tissue. Increases in this suggest swelling associated with injuries – consider compression of the trachea.

Thoracic and lumbar X-rays

- AP and lateral views are sufficient.
- **Assessing stability with the 3 columns theory**: the thoracic and lumbar vertebrae can be divided into three vertical columns (Fig. 2.6).

When 2 or all 3 columns are involved, the fracture is considered unstable.

- For example:
  - wedge fractures typically affect only the anterior column and so are stable;
  - burst fractures typically affect only the anterior and middle column, and so are potentially unstable;
  - major fractures/dislocation affect all columns and so are unstable.

Anterior column
Anterior longitudinal ligament and anterior two-thirds vertebral body.

Middle column
Posterior third vertebral body to posterior longitudinal ligament.

Posterior column
From the posterior longitudinal ligament pedicles to the tip of the spinous processes.

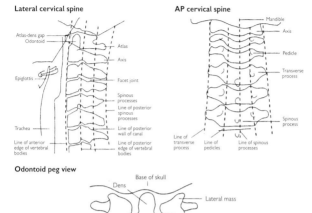

Fig. 2.5 Interpreting a lateral cervical spine X-ray. Reproduced from Wyatt J. et al. *Oxford Handbook of Emergency Medicine*, 3rd Edition, 2006, with permission from Oxford University Press.

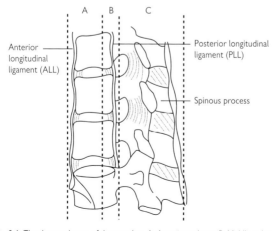

Fig. 2.6 The three columns of the vertebra. A. Anterior column; B. Middle column; C. Posterior column.

☠ **Penetrating neck injury**

The neck is divided into three zones, which is useful when describing injuries, predicting structures at risk of damage, and in determining management (see Fig. 2.7):
- Zone 1 = clavicles to cricoid cartilage.
- Zone 2 = cricoid to angle of mandible.
- Zone 3 = angle of mandible to skull base.

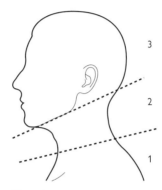

Fig. 2.7 The zones of the neck.

Breach of the platysma muscle is an indicator of serious penetrating trauma. However, wounds should only be explored by senior surgeons who are familiar with the anatomy, and proficient in head and neck surgery.

Presentation

Mechanism and predisposing factors
- Stabbing.
- Slashing.
- Gun shot wound (GSW).

Signs, symptoms and clinical findings
- Hoarse voice, stridor, haemoptysis or haematemesis (from direct airway injury or compression by expanding haematoma).
- Surgical emphysema in neck (laryngeal, oesophageal, or lung injury).
- Pneumothorax or haemothorax.
- External bleeding or expanding haematoma (vascular injury).
- Tachycardia or hypotension from hypovolaemic shock.
- Caroid bruit on auscultation.
- Neurological deficit, e.g. cerebrovascular accident (CVA) or reduced GCS from reduced cerebral perfusion or from spinal cord injury.

Management
- Assess for life threatening airway or breathing problems.
- Immobilize cervical spine if history of simultaneous blunt trauma or neurology.
- Oxygen 15 L.
- Direct pressure if any bleeding from wound.
- IV access (2× wide bore) and bloods including X match.
- IV sodium chloride 0.9% 250 mL boluses to maintain radial pulse.
- Urgent ENT, maxillofacial, or vascular surgeon input. Zone 1 injuries may also need cardiothoracic input.
- Portable CXR to exclude pneumothorax or haemothorax.
- Consider soft tissue lateral neck X-ray (if patient stable) for FB.
- Consider tetanus status and prophylactic IV antibiotics according to hospital policy.

Further management
- **Unstable patient:** immediate exploration in theatre.
- **Stable patient:** options include surgical exploration, angiography, Duplex ultrasound scan, contrast swallow investigations, or CT according to surgeons assessment.

Breathing

☻ **Assessment of breathing**

Assessment of breathing should take place after assessment of the airway and immobilization of the cervical spine. The aim of the primary survey is to identify life threatening chest injuries. All major trauma patients should receive 15 L oxygen via a non-rebreathing mask with a reservoir bag to optimize their inspired oxygen concentration.

Assessment

- **Assess the neck:** look for tracheal deviation, wounds, surgical emphysema, laryngeal crepitus, or distended neck veins. The cervical collar may need to be removed with MILS, whilst this is performed.
- **Fully expose the chest:** cut away all clothes and assess all areas of the anterior chest including the axillae and the top of the shoulders.
- **Count respiratory rate.**
- **Inspect:** look for deformity, bruising, abrasions, swelling, wounds, paradoxical movements of a flail and symmetrical chest expansion.
- **Palpate:** feel along the clavicles, sternum, and ribs for tenderness, crepitus, instability, or surgical emphysema in the soft tissues.
- **Percuss:** percuss bilaterally for hyper-resonance or dullness (this may not be easy in a busy Resuscitation room wearing gloves).
- **Auscultate** for bilateral air entry in the axilla, and upper and lower chest on each side.
- **Pulse oximetry.**
- **Check the back of the chest:** this may involve a gloved hand passed under the supine patient from the shoulders to the buttocks to exclude any injury. If the patient has no obvious life-threatening injuries on a primary survey, a log roll can be performed to directly visualize the posterior thorax. This is particularly important in patients with penetrating trauma, where wounds to the back may have been missed.

Investigations

Focused assessment with sonography for trauma (FAST)

Pericardial views on ultrasound can demonstrate pericardial fluid or cardiac tamponade.

Emergency ultrasound can also be used to assess for the presence of pneumothorax or haemothorax by a trained operator. During the abdominal scan hepatorenal and lienorenal views, the probe can be slid towards the patients head to visualize the diaphragm and lung on each side. Free fluid (e.g. haemothorax) is seen as a black stripe between the diaphragm and the lung.

Anterior thorax views in the 2nd or 3rd intercostal space in the mid-clavicular line may demonstrate a pneumothorax in a supine patient if one is present. The signs are an absence of 'lung sliding' and 'comet tail' artefacts. A negative scan does not exclude a pneumothorax as air may not have collected in this area.

Portable chest X-ray

CXR is not 100% reliable for pneumothorax in a supine patient as air will collect anteriorly. Subtle signs include hyperlucency over the liver or a 'deep sulcus sign', which is a sharply defined costophrenic angle and junction of the mediastinum with diaphragm, as it is outlined by air. Haemothorax will be seen as a whiter lung compared with the uninjured side if the patient is supine and fluid has collected posteriorly. The mediastinum may appear widened on a normal supine CXR, but should be investigated further if there is any suspicion of traumatic aortic disruption. Rib and clavicle fractures may be identified on a plain film, and indicate a high mechanism of injury to the chest.

Arterial blood gases

Blood gas sampling is important to assess the adequacy of oxygenation and need for invasive ventilation.

Echocardiogram

Cardiac contusion may cause changes in the ST segments or arrhythmias.

Computed tomography scan

Are especially useful in detecting pulmonary parenchymal changes and aortic injuries.

⑦ Mechanism of chest injury

Blunt
Chest injury can result from three mechanisms – direct blow causing contusion or perforation, crush injury, or a deceleration injury causing shearing. The most common mechanisms are RTC, assault, fall from height, sporting injury, or industrial crush injury.

Penetrating
Any wound between the neck and umbilicus may cause intrathoracic injury. The diaphragm moves up to the 5th intercostal space (nipple line in males) on expiration and, therefore, any wound between the nipple line and costal margin may be a chest or abdominal injury.

Blast lung
Blast waves from an explosion can cause injury as follows:
- **Primary:** disruption at sites where tissues of different density meet (e.g. air and lung mass) causing pulmonary contusion, pneumothorax, haemothorax, traumatic lung cysts, pneumomediastinum, or subcutaneous emphysema.
- **Secondary:** penetrating chest injury from fragments.
- **Tertiary:** chest wall injury from being thrown by the blast wave.

Failure of oxygenation or ventilation in trauma
Causes include:
- Pain from rib, spinal, or sternal fractures.
- Loss of integrity of chest wall affecting mechanics of respiration.
- Inadequate lung inflation due to pneumothorax or haemothorax.
- Damage to lung tissue, e.g. contusion.
- Diaphragmatic injury.
- Poor pulmonary perfusion from hypovolaemic shock.
- Reduced conscious level with hypoventilation.

☻ Life-threatening chest injuries

The clinical signs listed in Table 3.1 may help to differentiate isolated life-threatening chest injuries in the primary survey. Remember that the blood pressure may be low due to other sources of haemorrhage.

Table 3.1 Clinical signs of chest injuries

	Chest wall inspection	Percussion	Air entry	Blood pressure
Tension pneumothorax	Hyperexpanded	Hyperresonant	Reduced	May be decreased
Open pneumothorax	Wound	Hyperresonant	Reduced	Normal
Massive haemothorax	Reduced movement	Dull	Reduced	Decreased
Flail chest	Deformity	Often difficult as pain	Reduced	Normal or high
Cardiac tamponade	Possible wound	Normal	Normal	Decreased

Circulation

:☠: **Shock**

Shock is defined as 'inadequate tissue perfusion and oxygenation'.

Potential causes of shock in the trauma patient
- **Hypovolaemia:** loss of circulating volume, e.g. haemorrhage or burns.
- **Cardiogenic:** failure of the pump mechanism, e.g. cardiac contusion
- **Obstructive:** cardiac output is compromised by external compressive forces, e.g. tension pneumothorax or cardiac tamponade.
- **Neurogenic:** vasodilatation from loss of sympathetic outflow, e.g. spinal injury.

Hypovolaemic shock
Haemorrhage, defined as an acute loss of circulating blood volume, is the most common cause of shock in the trauma patient.

Potential sources of haemorrhage
- External bleeding.
- Chest.
- Abdomen and retroperitoneum.
- Pelvis.
- Femurs.

This can be remembered easily as 'blood on the floor and four more'.

Signs, symptoms and clinical findings
- Tachypnoea.
- Tachycardia (bradycardia is a late pre-terminal sign).
- Hypotension [systolic blood pressure (SBP < 90 mmHg)].
- Pallor and cold peripheries.
- Reduced conscious level.
- Reduced urinary output.
- ABG metabolic acidosis.

Grading of shock in adult patients
In a healthy adult patient the blood volume is approximately 7% of ideal body weight, e.g. a 70-kg patient has a circulating blood volume of approximately 5 L. The blood volume of a child is approximately 80 mL/kg.

The compensatory mechanisms evoked by shock (tachycardia and progressive vasoconstriction) are useful in determining the approximate amount of blood loss in a patient (see Table 4.1). Note that hypotension is a late sign.

Table 4.1 Clinical features of blood loss

Grade	Blood loss	Clinical features
I	Up to 750 mL <15%	Tachypnoea May have mild tachycardia
II	750–1500 mL 15–30%	Tachycardia >100 Narrowed pulse pressure Pallor
III	1500–2000 mL 30–40%	Hypotension Reduced GCS, confused or anxious
IV	>2000 mL >40%	May become bradycardic Marked hypotension Becoming unconscious

Pitfalls

There are several pitfalls that may lead to a gross over or underestimation of blood loss. These include:

- **The elderly:** who are less able to compensate for acute hypovolaemia as their sympathetic drive is reduced.
- **Medications:** e.g. beta blockers may prevent a tachycardia in response to blood loss.
- **Pacemakers:** pulse will not be altered by blood loss.
- **Hypothermia:** respiratory rate, pulse and blood pressure will be low regardless of blood loss.
- **Children:** will compensate well initially and then deteriorate catastrophically.
- **Pregnancy:** blood volume increases by up to 50% of normal so may only display minimal signs of shock with severe blood loss.
- **Athletes:** physiological responses to training means a larger blood volume and lower resting heart rate. Therefore, even a pulse of 90 may be a significant tachycardia in these patients.

Log-rolling

Patients with hypovolaemic shock from non-compressible haemorrhage should not be log-rolled. The movements of log-rolling can cause dislodgement of formed clots and allow further ongoing haemorrhage with cardiovascular collapse or cardiac arrest of the patient. A scoop stretcher or PAT slide can be used to transfer the patient off the spinal board or trolley. The back can be examined by running gloved hands down the back to check for haemorrhage or a 10–15° 'mini' log roll to examine first one half of the back and then the other half.

:☼: **Management of hypovolaemia**

Principles include control of haemorrhage, fluid resuscitation, and prevention of hypothermia and monitoring of response.

Haemorrhage control

External bleeding

The majority of external bleeding can be controlled by direct pressure and elevation. There will be rare occasions where a commercial tourniquet may be necessary to control limb haemorrhage.

Internal bleeding

- **Chest:** theatre.
- **Abdomen:** theatre.
- **Pelvis:** external splintage +/– theatre or embolization.
- **Femurs:** external splintage +/– theatre.

Principles of fluid resuscitation

What fluids?

- Initial fluid resuscitation should begin with the administration of a warmed crystalloid.
- Blood should be taken for X-match as soon as possible. Phone blood bank to let them know if the sample is urgent.
- Non-responders (who show no haemodynamic improvement with initial fluid administration) should receive urgent surgical input and O-negative blood.
- Transient responders (vital signs improve after fluids, but subsequently deteriorate due to ongoing haemorrhage) should receive urgent surgical input, and group-specific or O-negative blood.
- Rapid responders (vital signs stabilize permanently after fluids) normally require only crystalloid and can wait for fully cross-matched blood if required.

How much?

- In a patient with ongoing non-compressible haemorrhage, large volumes of fluid are thought to be associated with a poor outcome. Raising the blood pressure may dislodge clots resulting in further haemorrhage, and fluids dilute clotting factors and the oxygen carrying capacity of the blood.
- The aim is to administer sufficient fluids to maintain perfusion of the vital organs until the patient gets to theatre. In the normal adult patient, this means using boluses of 250 mL to maintain a systolic blood pressure of 80–90 mmHg, a radial pulse or a verbal response.
- The exceptions to this are patients with evidence of a head injury who require a higher BP to maintain cerebral perfusion pressure. The target BP in this case is 100 mmHg.

Options for vascular access (📖 Vascular access, p44)
- Peripheral venous cannulation.
- Intra-osseous access.
- Central venous cannulation, e.g. femoral, internal jugular, subclavian.
- Venous cut down, e.g. saphenous.

Massive transfusion

This is defined as 'replacement of the patients total blood volume in <24 h or acute administration of >50% estimated blood volume per hour'. Complications include hypothermia, dilutional thrombocytopenia, depletion of clotting factors, oxygen affinity changes, and hypocalcaemia.

Most hospitals have a policy for massive blood transfusion, which you should be familiar with. Check International Normalized Ratio (INR), activated partial thromboplastin time (APTT), platelets, and fibrinogen if patient is still under your care after first hour. Seek advice from haematology regarding administration of platelets, fresh frozen plasma, or cryoprecipitate.

Damage control surgery

Multiple injured trauma patients commonly die from a triad of coagulopathy, hypothermia, and acidosis, which forms a vicious circle. The shortest possible operation should be performed to control haemorrhage, prevent contamination and protect against further injury. This may include packing the abdominal cavity to stop bleeding, the use of shunts, and only temporarily closing the abdomen or leaving it open. The patient is then transferred to the critical care unit for aggressive correction of coagulopathy and rewarming, before a definitive surgical procedure at a later date (usually 24–48 h).

Prevention of hypothermia

Every effort should be made to ensure the patient does not become cold which will worsen acidosis and coagulopathy. Check the patient's temperature (this is often omitted if the patient is immobilized in head blocks for a suspected cervical spine injury). Consider an oesophageal temperature probe.

Keep warm externally with blankets and a bear hugger. Fluids should be kept in a warming cupboard in the Resuscitation room prior to administration. Use of a warming system around the giving set is another option, but will slow the rate of administration.

Monitor response

The following should be monitored:
- Respiratory rate, O_2 saturation.
- ECG for pulse, BP.
- Catheterize for hourly urine output.
- GCS.
- ABG for acidosis, lactate, or Hb.

☠ **Vascular access**

Peripheral venous cannulation

This is the first choice of vascular access. Flow rates through venflons depend on the following:

• Diameter of venflon (flow proportional to r^4).
• Length of venflon (flow inversely proportional to length).
• Viscosity of fluid.
• Pressure (increase flow by raising height of fluid bag or external pressure).

A comparison of the flow rates through a BD Venflon™ Pro are as follows:

• **Pink 20G:** 13 mL/min.
• **Green 18G:** 103 mL/min.
• **Grey 16G:** 236 mL/min.
• **Orange 14G:** 270 mL/min.

Therefore, the largest possible venflon should be inserted in each antecubital fossa. Only in extreme situations should the external jugular vein of the neck be used. Make sure you secure the cannula and tubing to the skin, and document insertion in the notes.

Intra-osseous

This is the second option if peripheral venous access is unsuccessful on two or more attempts in a shocked patient, or may be the first option if the shocked patient has no obvious peripheral veins, or has extensive burns.

The intra-osseous (IO) space has a resting pressure of approximately 35/25 mmHg and, therefore, compared with the venous pressure of 0–10 mmHg, there is high resistance to flow. This can be overcome by flushing the IO access initially to open the vascular channels in the bone marrow and then using pressure on the fluid bag, or using a 50 mL syringe and 3-way tap to bolus fluids. Manufacturers of IO devices quote that once the drug or fluid has entered the IO space, circulation times are comparable to traditional intravenous access.

All drugs that can be given via the IV route may be given by the IO route.

The IO route can be painful and, therefore, local anaesthetic may need to be used subcutaneously prior to insertion of the IO needle and via the intra-osseous route prior to fluid administration.

The IO access can be left *in situ* until alternative large peripheral access is obtained or up to 24 h.

Contraindications: fracture of bone selected for insertion, inability to locate landmarks, compromised extremity, infection at site of insertion, underlying bone disease, e.g. tumour or osteoporosis.

Sites
- Anterior surface of the tibia 2 cm inferior and medial to tibial tuberosity.
- Humeral head at site of greater tubercle.
- Sternum: only if commercial device designed for this purpose.

Complications: extravasation, haematoma, compartment syndrome, bone injury, skin infection, or osteomyelitis.

There are a number of commercial products on the market for IO access. These include the standard COOK IO needle (paediatric only, Fig. 4.1), FAST-1 (adult only), EZ-IO (adult or paediatric needles), and BIG (paediatric or adult versions available). Familiarize yourself with the IO needles (and manufacturers information) available in your Resuscitation room.

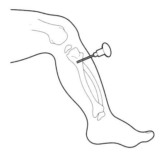

Fig. 4.1 Tibial intra-osseous access. Reproduced from Wyatt *et al.* (2006), with permission from Oxford University Press.

Venous cut down

This technique requires time and surgical skill so is only useful for experienced practitioners. The long saphenous vein is located 2 cm above and anterior to the medial malleolus of the ankle.
- Locate landmarks and sterilize site with povidone-iodine or antiseptic solution. Use an aseptic technique with sterile gloves.
- Use local anaesthetic subcutaneously in a conscious patient at the site of incision.
- Make a 2.5 cm transverse incision until the vessel is located. Gently separate the vein from any accompanying structures using a haemostat (Fig. 4.2).
- Pass two 2-0 sutures beneath the vein and tie the distal one with two long strands to apply traction to the vessel.

• Make a small incision in the vein and insert a large bore plastic catheter (venflon) proximally. Tie the proximal suture to secure the vessel around the catheter. Flush with sodium chloride 0.9% to ensure patency and commence infusion of fluids.
• Close the incision with interrupted sutures. Apply a sterile dressing and tape.

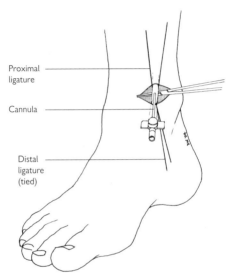

Proximal
ligature

Cannula

Distal
ligature
(tied)

Fig. 4.2 Cut down access to long saphenous vein. Reproduced from Allman et al. (2005), with permission from Oxford University Press.

Complications: haematoma, perforation of vein, venous thrombosis, nerve damage.

Central venous cannulation

Insertion of central lines is a difficult technique with a high incidence of complications. Narrow bore lines are not ideal for the rapid administration of fluids and central access is, therefore, a last resort option.

Ultrasound guidance should be used for all central line insertions to reduce the risk of complications. Veins will be larger, more oval, compressible (unless full of thrombus), the diameter will change with valsalva or respiration, and Doppler waveform analysis may further differentiate a vein from an artery.

Prior to access the skin is cleaned around the site, the vein is identified using an ultrasound probe and local anaesthetic is infiltrated subcutaneously if the patient is conscious.

A Seldinger technique is used at all sites, which involves inserting a hollow needle attached to a syringe into the vein until there is free aspiration of venous blood. A flexible guidewire is threaded through the needle and the needle is removed. A tapered dilator and then the plastic cannula are inserted over the guidewire and gently advanced into the vein. The guidewire is then removed, the cannula is checked for free aspiration, is flushed with sodium chloride 0.9% and sutured in place. A dressing is applied and CXR requested for IJ or SC access.

Contraindications: anticoagulants or bleeding disorders, no previous experience in insertion.

Complications: arterial puncture, haematoma, haemothorax or pneumothorax, air embolism, cardiac arrhythmia.

Femoral vein
- Patient is supine with leg slightly abducted.
- The femoral vein lies just medial to the femoral artery and just inferior to the inguinal ligament.

Internal jugular vein

Patient is supine with a head down tilt. It is virtually impossible to perform in the neutral position (with MILS, and removal of head blocks and collar) if the cervical spine has not been cleared and, therefore, may not be a viable option.

The vein is identified lateral to the carotid artery at the centre of the triangle formed by the two lower heads of the sternomastoid muscle and the clavicle. The needle is advanced at a 45° angle towards the ipsilateral nipple (Fig. 4.3).

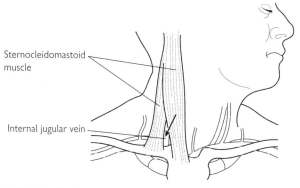

Sternocleidomastoid muscle

Internal jugular vein

Fig. 4.3 Internal jugular access.

Subclavian vein (infraclavicular approach)

• Patient is supine with a head down tilt.
• The site of insertion is 1 cm inferior to the mid-clavicular point, advancing below the clavicle, and medially towards the sternal notch.
• This approach carries the highest risk of pneumothorax. If one side of the chest already has an injury or chest drain *in situ*, use this side of the neck for insertion.
• See Fig. 4.4.

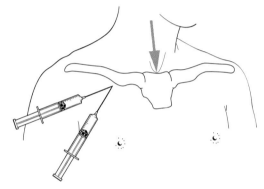

Fig. 4.4 Subclavian access. Reproduced from Myerson et al. (2006), with permission from Oxford University Press.

References

Allman, K., *et al.* (2005) *Emergencies in Anaesthesia*. Oxford: Oxford University Press.

Myerson, G., *et al.* (2006) *Emergencies in Cardiology*, 2006. Oxford: Oxford University Press.

Wyatt, J., *et al.* (2006) *Oxford Handbook of Emergency Medicine*, 3rd edn. Oxford: Oxford University Press.

☣ **Emergency department thoracotomy**

This extremely rare procedure should only be performed by an operator who has been trained to perform the procedure and has previous experience.

Indications

- Penetrating injury to chest or upper abdomen, e.g. stab wound.
- **With** witnessed cardiac arrest with signs of life in the last 10 min.
- **And** suspected cardiac tamponade.

There is no current role for emergency thoracotomy after blunt trauma.

Clam shell thoracotomy (Fig. 4.5)

- Call for senior help and cardiothoracic support (this may be a surgical consultant or senior registrar), but do not wait for it to arrive to start procedure.
- Continue ALS protocol with cardiac compressions, rapid intravenous fluids, and ask the anaesthetist to simultaneously intubate the patient and provide positive pressure ventilation.
- Rapidly clean the skin with iodine or alcohol-based solution. Using a scalpel make bilateral thoracostomy incisions in the 4th or 5th intercostal spaces anterior to the mid-axillary line, into the pleural space. If a tension pneumothorax is released and the patient has return of spontaneous circulation, stop and reassess.
- Extend the incisions on either side to the midline, following the intercostal muscle to the sternum. Stop ventilating the patient at the point of incision to avoid a lung laceration.
- Use robust scissors to divide the sternum.

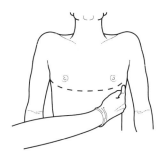

Fig. 4.5 Incision for clam shell thoracotomy.

- Use manual retraction by a double-gloved assistant or use rib retractors to spread the ribs open.
- Identify the heart, pick up the pericardium with forceps, and cut longitudinally in the midline through the anterior pericardium avoiding the phrenic nerve. Evacuate any blood from the pericardial sac. This will allow return of cardiac output if there is an isolated cardiac tamponade.
- Identify any wounds to the heart and place a finger on any defect to apply direct pressure. For larger wounds a clamped Foley urinary catheter can be inserted into the hole with the balloon inflated once inside the chamber and gentle traction applied to occlude the hole.
- Bi-manual internal cardiac massage can be performed by compressing the heart between two flat hands, front and back.
- If the heart is fibrillating, use internal defibrillation paddles at 5J shock per cycle according to ALS guidelines. If these are not available, remove retraction, approximate the chest wall and defibrillate externally using a routine charge.
- Continue fluid resuscitation (blood or crystalloid IV) and ALS guidelines until arrival of a senior.

☠ **Pelvic fractures**

Pelvic fractures are one of the sources of life-threatening internal haemorrhage, which should be detected on the primary survey. Bleeding can occur from the fracture site, the surrounding soft tissues, and the pelvic blood vessels disrupted at the time of injury.

Presentation
- RTC occupant, pedestrian, or motorcyclist.
- Crush type injury, e.g. horse rolls on rider.
- Falls from height.
- Elderly osteoporotic patients after simple fall.

Signs, symptoms, and clinical findings
- **Signs of hypovolaemic shock.**
- **Evidence of pelvic injury.**
- Pain in groin, hips, genitals, or lower back (SI joint).
  - Swelling, bruising, or deformity to the iliac crests or pubic symphysis.
- Wounds over the pelvis suggestive of open fractures.
- Unequal leg length, excluding fractures in that extremity.
- External bleeding from rectum, vagina, or the urethra in males.
- **Signs of urethral injury.**
  - Perineal bruising, blood at the meatus, high-riding prostate on per rectum (PR) examination.

Investigations
- FBC, clotting, U&E, group and save (G&S)/ X-match as minimum.
- Initially, portable AP pelvis radiograph (Fig. 4.6) and CXR to look for associated injuries.
- A CT pelvis when the patient is stable gives most information.

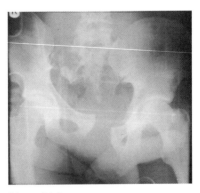

Fig. 4.6 Vertical sheat pelvic fracture.

Management

- ABC and oxygen.
- IV access and bloods including X-match.
- Administer 250 mL boluses of 0.9% saline to maintain SBP >90 mmHg.
- **Do not spring or palpate the pelvis:** this will move the fracture site and dislodge clots resulting in further internal haemorrhage. Be guided by the mechanism of injury, symptoms, or signs to suggest a possible pelvic fracture, and treat as such.
- If a pelvic splint has been applied pre-admission, leave in place, and await X-rays.
- **Apply a commercial pelvic splint** onto bare skin at the level of the greater trochanters to stabilize the fracture. If no commercial splint is available use a sheet tied around the pelvis.
- Internally rotate legs and secure ankles with figure of eight bandage to prevent movement of hips.
- **Avoid log-rolling the patient** if at all possible: use a scoop stretcher to transfer or slide the patient on a pat-slide board.
- Obtain a portable X-ray of the pelvis. If this is normal and the patient is normovolaemic with minimal pain, the pelvic splint can be gently released with palpation of the pelvis. If there is any suspicion of injury, a CT should be performed presuming the patient is stable.
- Refer pelvic fractures urgently to a pelvic/orthopaedic surgeon.

Complications

Urethral injury
- **Do not** insert urinary catheter if any bleeding at external urethra.
- Urgently refer to Urology for further investigation of the urethral injury and potential suprapubic catheter.

Open fractures
- Carry a mortality of 50%.
- Control external haemorrhage with direct pressure.
- Remove any gross contamination and irrigate with 0.9% saline.
- Cover wounds with sterile Betadine dressing.
- Ensure covered for tetanus and IV antibiotic prophylaxis.

Concurrent injuries
- Include bowel perforation, head injury, chest injury, and diaphragmatic rupture.
- Paralytic ileus is a common complication in the days following major pelvic fracture associated with bleeding, necessitating a nasogastric (NG) tube.

Management of hypovolaemia in patients with pelvic fractures

Apply an external pelvic splint (Fig. 4.7)

↓

Fluid resuscitation
250-mL boluses crystalloid fluid, to maintain
SBP >90 mmHg.
Follow with O negative or X-matched blood
AS SOON AS AVAILABLE
Follow hospital massive transfusion protocol to prevent coagulopathy,
and adminster blood, cryoprecipitate, fresh frozen plasma,
and platelets on advice of haematologist.

↓

Exclude other sources of haemorrhage
including chest, abdomen, femurs, and occult external bleeding,
and manage accordingly.

↓

Continued hypovolaemia requires emergency **angiography for
embolization** of bleeding pelvic vessels.

↓

Continued hypovolaemia (or angiography not available) may require a
laparatomy to ligate bleeding vessels or for retroperitoneal packing –
senior Trauma team members must decide with consultant surgeons.

↓

Investigations
FBC, clotting, X-match
Portable AP pelvis and CXR
FAST scan
ABG
CT angiogram

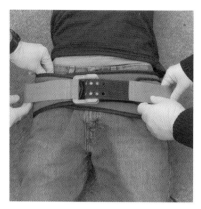

Fig. 4.7 SAM splint. Reproduced with permission of SAM Medical products® www.sammedical.com
Note: Splint should be applied directly to skin.

:⚙: Femoral shaft fracture

Presentation
Mechanism and predisposing factors
- RTC occupant, pedestrian, or motorcyclist.
- Falls from height.

Signs, symptoms, and clinical findings
- Pain in thigh or hip.
- Swelling, bruising, tenderness, or deformity to thigh.
- Wound if open fracture (may be in-out or have protruding bone).
- Shortening of affected limb +/– external rotation.

Investigations
AP and lateral X-rays of the whole femur (including hip and knee) are required.

Management
- ABC.
- IV access and bloods, including X-match 4 units.
- IV analgesia, e.g. morphine titrated to response.
- IV fluids to maintain systolic BP >90 mmHg.
- Check distal pulses and sensation.
- Application of traction splint, e.g. Thomas splint.
- Plain X-ray femur AP and lateral.
- Refer to Orthopaedics for operative fixation (usually proximal or retrograde intramedullary nailing).

Analgesia
- Intravenous morphine or ketamine.
- Femoral nerve block.
- Traction and splintage.

Open femoral fractures
- Control external haemorrhage with direct pressure.
- Remove any gross contamination and irrigate with sodium chloride 0.9%.
- Cover wounds with sterile saline soaked or Betadine dressing.
- Ensure covered for tetanus and IV antibiotic prophylaxis.
- Will require wound debridement and external fixation in theatre followed by delayed definitive treatment (proximal or retrograde intramedullary nailing following removal of external fixation).

Complications
- Haemorrhage.
- Neurovascular injury.
- Fat embolism.
- Compartment syndrome.
- Infection in open fracture.

Femoral nerve block (Fig. 4.8)

- Avoid in patients who you are concerned may develop compartment syndrome, as this may go undetected.
- The femoral nerve is located 1 cm lateral to the femoral artery, just below the inguinal ligament.
- Ultrasound or a nerve stimulator may be useful to identify the correct site.
- Clean the skin using povidone-iodine or antiseptic solution.
- Use 10–20 mL of 1% lidocaine or 0.25% bupivacaine in adults.
- Insert the needle at a 45° angle to a depth of approximately 3 cm. If paraesthesia or severe pain occurs, the needle has penetrated the nerve and should be withdrawn slightly before injection to prevent neuronal damage.
- Aspirate to check for inadvertent arterial or venous puncture prior to injection.
- Nerve block lasts approximately 4–6 h if using lidocaine.
- Most effectively undertaken with the use of a nerve stimulator.

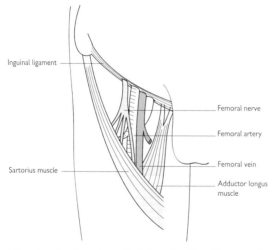

Fig. 4.8 Anatomy for a femoral nerve block. Reproduced from Myerson et al. (2006) with permission from Oxford University Press.

Application of Thomas splint (Fig. 4.9)

- Measure the circumference of the uninjured thigh and select a splint with the appropriate ring size and length (making allowance for swelling).
- Wrap the ring in cotton wool and slide a length of tubigrip or commercially available sling along the poles of the splint which will support the leg.
- Ensure the patient has received adequate analgesia, e.g. morphine plus femoral nerve block, and provide manual longitudinal traction on the injured leg from the heel.
- Apply the adhesive foam to the skin over the malleoli and proximally up each side of the leg. Bandage the leg from ankle to mid thigh with a crepe bandage.
- Slide the splint over the leg until it is resting against the perineum. Ensure it is an appropriate size and that the genitalia are not under pressure from the ring. Pad with cotton wool to prevent sores.
- Tie the cords from the heel end of the skin traction to the end of the splint. Insert two tongue depressors (taped together) between the cords and twist until tight. Ensure manual traction is maintained until the cords are secured.
- Check distal pulses and sensation.
- Obtain a repeat X-ray.

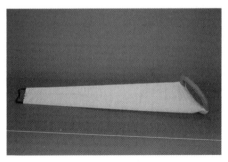

Fig. 4.9 Thomas splint.

Reference

Myerson, G., et al. (2006) *Emergencies in Cardiology*. Oxford: Oxford University Press.

Thoracic trauma

☠ Tension pneumothorax

Tension pneumothorax results from a breach in the lung pleura, which functions as a one-way valve, so air can enter the pleural cavity on inspiration, but not exit on expiration.

This leads to ipsilateral lung collapse; mediastinal deviation with compression of the great vessels obstructing venous return to the heart; and contralateral lung compression. It is rare in non-ventilated spontaneously breathing patients.

Presentation

Mechanism and predisposing factors

- Penetrating or blunt chest trauma.
- Iatrogenic following central line insertion.
- Barotrauma from positive high pressure ventilation.
- Ventilated patients with an undiagnosed simple pneumothorax.

Signs, symptoms, and clinical findings

- **In awake patients:** progressive chest pain, respiratory distress, tachypnoea, hypoxia, and tachycardia. If untreated hypotension, bradycardia, and cardiac arrest with PEA will result.
- **In ventilated patients:** rapid onset hypoxia, high ventilation pressures, and hypotension.
- Localizing signs of ipsilateral hyperexpansion and hypomobility of the chest wall, hyper-resonance to percussion, and reduced breath sounds on auscultation.
- Distended neck veins and a deviated trachea are rare in practice.

Investigations

The diagnosis should be clinical. A CXR should not be requested on a deteriorating patient with a suspected tension pneumothorax. However, in the absence of haemodynamic compromise in cases where the diagnosis is in doubt, it may be appropriate to wait for the results of an emergency CXR prior to intervention (Fig. 5.1).

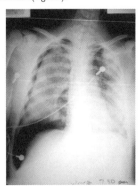

Fig. 5.1 X-ray of right tension pneumothorax.

Needle thoracocentesis

- This should be performed immediately in any patient with significant respiratory compromise +/– haemodynamic instability if there is clinical suspicion of tension pneumothorax.
- Attach a 10-mL syringe to a 14G venflon.
- Identify the 2nd intercostal space in the mid-clavicular line on the affected side of the chest.
- Insert the venflon at this site perpendicular to the skin over the top of the 3rd rib (to avoid the neurovascular bundle) aspirating the syringe as advanced. Rapid aspiration of air confirms the diagnosis.
- Remove the needle and syringe, leaving the plastic cannula *in situ* open to air, and dispose of sharps safely.
- Urgently re-assess the patient's clinical status.
- If improved obtain a portable CXR and prepare for rapid chest drain insertion.

Failure of needle thoracocentesis

This may be due to:
- Incorrect initial diagnosis.
- Kinking of the cannula.
- Plugging with tissue or blood.
- Inadequate length to penetrate parietal pleura.
- A larger air leak than can be drained by the narrow bore of the cannula.
- Loculated tension pneumothorax.

Thoracostomy

- In the situation where the diagnosis of tension pneumothorax is in no doubt, but the patient is still deteriorating despite needle thoracocentesis, thoracostomy is appropriate.
- Using a scalpel make a 3–4 cm incision in the lateral chest wall in the 5th intercostal space anterior to the mid-axillary line (where a chest drain is usually sited). Create a passage through the intercostal muscles using Spencer Wells forceps. Insert a gloved finger to penetrate the pleura and expand the opening to release air from the pleural space.
- Thoracostomy should be followed immediately by chest drain insertion and CXR.

Chest drain insertion

All patients who have had needle thoracocentesis or decompression of a tension pneumothorax to a simple pneumothorax should have a chest drain inserted at the earliest opportunity.

Pitfalls

- Misdiagnosis of tension pneumothorax in the presence of pulmonary contusion, haemothorax, large simple pneumothorax, or gastrothorax.
- Failure of needle thoracocentesis.
- Tension pneumothorax with a large air leak requiring more than one chest drain.

☼ Simple pneumothorax

A simple pneumothorax is a collection of air in the pleural space without clinical or radiological features of tension.

Presentation

Mechanism and predisposing factors
- Penetrating chest trauma, e.g. GSW or stabbing.
- Blunt chest injury with rib fracture or contusion.
- Blast injury.
- Iatrogenic following central line insertion.

Signs, symptoms, and clinical findings
- Short of breath (SOB) and pleuritic chest pain.
- May be overlying subcutaneous emphysema, local tenderness, or crepitus suggesting rib fractures.
- Localizing signs of reduced chest movement, with hyper-resonance to percussion and decreased air entry on affected side.
- Localized wheeze or crepitations.

Investigations

Emergency department ultrasound
Absent 'lung sliding' or absent 'comet tails' suggests the possibility of a pneumothorax.

CXR
Supine trauma CXR may miss small pneumothoraces as air will lay anterior in the pleural space. Subtle signs include a more radiolucent hemithorax on the affected side, a deep lateral costophrenic angle ('deep sulcus sign'), or a film of air around the cardiac shadow.

CT scan
CT is highly sensitive for pneumothorax. Very small pneumothoraces detectable only on CT scan may not require a chest drain in a spontaneously ventilating patient. Senior advice should be sought.

Management
- Supplementary oxygen, IV access, and IV analgesia.
- The majority of traumatic simple pneumothoraces will require insertion of chest drain on the affected side.

:☺: Open pneumothorax

Open pneumothorax results from a defect in the chest wall creating a communication between the pleural space and the external environment. If the opening is greater than two-thirds the diameter of the trachea, air will preferentially pass through the defect on inspiration following the path of least resistance to equilibrate atmospheric and intrathoracic pressures.

Presentation

Mechanism and predisposing factors
Penetrating chest wall trauma, e.g. GSW or stabbing.

Signs, symptoms, and clinical findings
- As for simple pneumothorax, but with a penetrating chest wall injury, which may be bubbling.
- Don't forget to check the back of the patient to avoid missing any wounds.

Investigations

As for simple pneumothorax.

Management

- Close defect with a commercial device, e.g. Asherman® chest seal or three-sided dressing to allow a flutter-valve effect, so the dressing will occlude the wound during inhalation, but during exhalation air can escape from the pleural space.
- Insertion of chest drain remote from the wound, at the usual site.
- Observe closely to identify any developing tension pneumothorax.
- Intravenous antibiotics as prophylaxis for wound infection.
- Senior surgical review of the patient.
- Definitive cardiothoracic surgery will be required to close the chest wall defect and identify any intrathoracic injury.

☠ Haemothorax

A haemothorax is a collection of blood in the pleural space as a result of injury to the lung parenchyma, pulmonary hilum, great vessels, chest wall, diaphragm, or a direct cardiac laceration.

Massive haemothorax is defined as more than 1500 mL of blood or one-third of the patient's blood volume in the pleural cavity.

Small haemothoraces may not be clinically detectable.

Presentation

Mechanism and predisposing factors
Penetrating; blunt; or blast injury.

Signs, symptoms and clinical findings
- Non-specific signs of penetrating chest injury, external bruising or swelling, or fractured ribs with crepitus.
- Tachypnoea and hypoxia.
- Localizing signs of hypomobility of chest wall, dull to percussion, reduced breath sounds on affected side.
- Tachycardia and hypotension from internal haemorrhage.

Investigations

CXR

The erect chest film demonstrates a classical fluid level, but takes approximately 500 mL of blood to obliterate the costophrenic angle. Haemothorax is difficult to diagnose on the supine trauma CXR with no fluid level as blood lies on the posterior chest wall causing diffuse opacification of the hemithorax (see Fig. 5.2). The differential diagnosis includes pulmonary contusion.

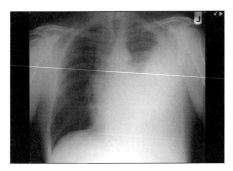

Fig. 5.2 X-ray of left haemothorax.

FAST scan

Emergency ultrasound may detect fluid/haemothorax above the diaphragm on upper quadrant views, but is difficult in the presence of pneumothorax or subcutaneous emphysema.

CT scan
- Emergency CT scan may be performed in haemodynamically stable patients.
- Significant haemothoraces should be drained and discussed with the Cardiothoracic team.
- Sub-clinical tiny haemothoraces detectable only on CT usually require no further action, but will need a follow up CXR to ensure no further expansion.

Management
- Oxygen, emergency intravenous access × 2 and send blood for cross-match.
- Commence infusion of crystalloid fluid or O-negative blood if the patient is hypotensive, using boluses of 250 mL until patient has SBP >90 mmHg.
- Chest drain insertion: >32 Fr for adults in order to drain blood from pleural cavity without clotting. Consider autotransfusion.
- Thoracotomy may be indicated if chest tube output is >1500 mL stat or >200 mL/h. Urgent cardiothoracic referral is advised.

Complications
- Hypovolaemic shock and death.
- Empyema from infected retained blood or non-sterile chest drain insertion.

Pitfalls
Always obtain reliable wide bore intravenous access prior to the insertion of a chest drain for massive haemothorax, or sudden decompression may result in haemodynamic collapse and inability to identify access.

☠ Flail chest

A flail chest is defined as a fracture of two or more ribs in two or more places. This results in an area of chest wall losing bony continuity with the thoracic cage and compromising mechanical ventilation. A flail segment is associated with significant injury to the underlying lung and pulmonary contusion.

A flail chest causes deterioration of the patient by the following means:
- Pain from multiple rib fractures preventing inspiratory effort.
- An underlying pulmonary contusion.
- Paradoxical movement of the chest wall reducing tidal volume.

Presentation
Mechanism and predisposing factors
Blunt injury or compression of the chest, e.g. crush.

Signs, symptoms and clinical findings
- Chest wall swelling, fractured ribs with crepitus.
- Reduced movement of chest on injured side, secondary to pain.
- Paradoxical movement may not be immediately apparent as splinting will initially occur from chest wall muscle spasm.
- Tachypnoea and hypoxia.

Investigations
CXR
Beware CXR may not demonstrate all fractures reliably.

CT scan
To identify underlying lung injury.

Management
- Supplementary oxygen.
- Intravenous analgesia.
- Judicious fluid replacement to prevent overloading of the injured lung.
- ABG to determine the need for RSI and mechanical ventilation.
- Contact ICU for advice regarding on-going management, e.g. analgesia and need for ventilation. Most patients with a flail chest require the minimum of high dependency unit (HDU) care.
- Operative stabilization of fractures is rarely performed.

Complications
- Respiratory failure.
- Underlying lung injury.
- Pneumonia.

Pitfalls

- Beware the posterior flail undetected when the patient is supine or the large anterior flail chest where chest wall movements appear symmetrical.
- Anterior and lateral paradoxical movements of the chest wall may not be seen when standing next to the patient: eyeball the supine patient from the end of the bed (Fig. 5.3).

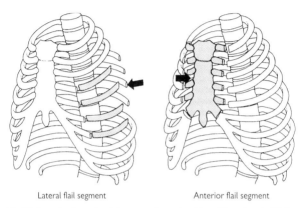

| Lateral flail segment | Anterior flail segment |

Fig. 5.3 Lateral and anterior flail segment. Reproduced from Wyatt J. *et al.* (2006) with permission from Oxford University Press.

Reference

Wyatt, J., *et al.* (2006) *Oxford Handbook of Emergency Medicine*, 3rd edn. Oxford: Oxford University Press.

☠ Cardiac tamponade

Injury that causes haemorrhage into the pericardial sac, compromising ventricular filling, and cardiac output will ultimately lead to cardiac arrest unless treated.

Presentation

Mechanism and predisposing factors

- Penetrating trauma, e.g. stab wounds or GSW to chest or abdomen (anterior, posterior, or lateral).
- Blunt chest wall trauma.

Signs, symptoms, and clinical findings

- Hypotension with penetrating chest or abdominal injuries, and other sources of life-threatening haemorrhage excluded.
- Beck's triad: distended neck veins, muffled heart sounds and hypotension. Do not over-emphasize these traditional signs as neck veins are often not distended because of hypovolaemia and heart sounds are difficult to auscultate in a busy Resuscitation room.
- Kussmaul's sign: rise in JVP on inspiration or pulsus paradoxus – reduction of SBP by more than 10 mmHg on inspiration are both subtle signs.
- PEA cardiac arrest.

Investigations

- FAST ultrasound scan (USS) demonstrates pericardial fluid, right ventricular collapse on sub-xiphoid view, and distended non-compressible IVC on abdominal views.
- ECG shows a low amplitude trace.

Immediate management

- Do not remove any penetrating objects, e.g. knife.
- Oxygen, 2× large bore IV access.
- IV fluids to maintain SBP ~90 mmHg maximum.
- Cardiac monitoring.
- Urgently seek cardiothoracic opinion. If not on site, call the General Surgery team, whilst contacting the tertiary referral centre.
- Call Anaesthetics/ICU and alert theatres.

If patient arrests

- Consider pericardiocentesis.
- Consider emergency department thoracotomy (see 📖 Emergency department thoracotomy, p50).

Pitfalls

Pericardiocentesis is often ineffective as clotted pericardial blood cannot be aspirated via the needle.

Pericardiocentesis

- Call for urgent senior cardiothoracic or general surgical assistance.
- Attach a 15-cm over-the-needle catheter to a 50-mL syringe.
- Use povidone-iodine or an alcohol wipe to sterilize the skin.
- Puncture the skin one fingers breadth inferior and to the left of the xiphisternum, and advance the needle at a 45° angle in all planes towards the tip of the left scapula.
- Monitor the ECG and aspirate as the needle is advanced. Any arrhythmia or ST segment changes indicate the needle needs to be withdrawn slightly.
- Withdraw as much blood as possible from the pericardial sac. If no further blood can be aspirated or ECG changes occur, stop, and secure the catheter in place.
- Reassess the patient and obtain urgent surgical input if successful.

Complications include aspiration of ventricular blood, arrhythmia, pneumothorax, myocardial injury, or penetration of the great vessels.

⑦ Chest drain insertion

Indications
- After needle decompression of suspected tension pneumothorax.
- To drain simple or open pneumothorax.
- To drain haemothorax.

Landmarks
4th or 5th intercostal space, anterior to mid-axillary line on affected side of hemi-thorax. Aim for the area within the 'safe triangle' bordered by the anterior border of latissiumus dorsi, the lateral border of pectoralis major, a line superior to the horizontal level of the nipple, and an apex in the axilla (Fig. 5.4).

Preparation
- Explain procedure to patient and obtain verbal consent if awake.
- Ensure patient is breathing oxygen, with full monitoring, and has 2 × IV access.
- If the patient is awake they will require titrated IV morphine prior to this painful procedure.
- Ensure all equipment is prepared and an assistant is available to help you.
- Prepare local anaesthetic, e.g. 1% lidocaine 10 mL.
- Set up the chest drain bottle with a water seal.
- Re-examine the patient, and any CXR or CT scan to confirm the side of the chest requiring a chest drain.

Procedure
- Abduct the arm on the affected side fully so the arm is behind the head.
- Wear a sterile gown and gloves. A face shield and eye protection is also advisable against splashes.
- Locate your landmarks on the patient. Clean the skin with antiseptic around the site of insertion and cover with sterile drapes.
- Generously infiltrate 1% lidocaine under the skin and over the 5th or 6th rib perpendicularly down to the pleural space (aspirating as the needle advances to avoid injection into a vessel).
- Remove any trocar from the chest drain and use the largest size that will easily pass through the ribs (24–32FG).
- Make a 3–4 cm incision in the line of the ribs, and use blunt dissection with Spencer Wells forceps to open the tissues over the 5th or 6th rib down to the pleural space. Enlarge the incision for access if required.
- Puncture the pleura with your finger, occasionally this is done with the forceps. This may lead to a release of air or blood on respiration. Immediately insert a gloved finger into the pleural cavity and sweep around the walls to ensure there are no adhesions. Be careful of rib fractures that may puncture your glove or finger!
- Insert the chest drain directed to the apex and posteriorly, ensuring that all drainage holes are within the pleural cavity. Connect the drain to an underwater seal drainage bottle and ensure it is 'swinging' with respiration.

- Recheck the patients clinical condition and auscultate the chest for bilateral air entry. A painful drain may indicate it has been advanced too far and is abutting the lung or mediastinum – withdraw a couple of centimetres and reassess.
- Secure the drain in place by using one suture to hold the drain in place and another to close the hole around the tube. Cover the site with a transparent dressing and tape.
- Obtain a CXR to confirm the tube position – if the tube has been inserted too far, pull back slightly and re-secure in place.
- Ensure the underwater seal drainage bottle is below the level of the patient. Avoid clamping the tube.
- Immediate complications include laceration to intrathoracic or intra-abdominal organs, damage to intercostal nerves, or vessels, extrathoracic chest tube placement, subcutaneous emphysema at site, chest tube kinking, or dislodging.

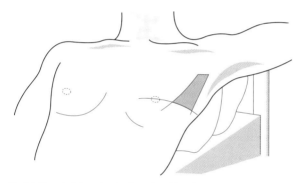

Fig. 5.4 Chest drain insertion site. Reproduced from Longmore *et al.* (2007), with permission from Oxford University Press.

Referral to thoracic surgeon
Referral is indicated if:
- Chest tube drains >1500 mL blood immediately or 200 mL/h (ongoing internal haemorrhage).
- Persistent continuous bubbling of air through underwater drain (may indicate rupture of tracheobronchial tree or significant lung injury).

Reference
Longmore M *et al.* (2007) *Oxford Handbook of Clinical Medicine*, 7th Edition. Oxford: Oxford University Press.

☼: Tracheobronchial injury

Presentation
Mechanism and predisposing factors
- Blunt neck trauma.
- Deceleration injury.
- Penetrating trauma, e.g. stab wounds, or GSW to neck or chest.

Signs, symptoms, and clinical findings
- Airway obstruction and respiratory distress.
- Bronchial injury: haemoptysis, subcutaneous emphysema to neck and chest, tension pneumothorax, or a pneumothorax with a large air leak after chest drain insertion.

Investigations
- CXR: pneumothorax, subcutaneous emphysema.
- Bronchoscopy by experienced anaesthetist or cardiothoracic surgeons.

Immediate management
- Oxygen, monitoring, and IV access.
- Urgent senior anaesthetic input to control airway. The patient may require main stem bronchial intubation with one lung ventilation or a tracheostomy.
- Urgent cardiothoracic review.
- An additional chest drain may be required if there is a large air leak with one chest drain.

Pitfalls
Difficult intubation and airway control due to distorted anatomy.

☼ Laryngeal injury

Presentation

Mechanism and predisposing factors
- Blunt neck trauma, e.g. horse rider impacting with branch.
- Penetrating trauma, e.g. stab wounds or GSW to neck.

Signs, symptoms, and clinical findings
- Airway obstruction and respiratory distress.
- Laryngeal injury: hoarse voice, haemoptysis, palpable crepitus over larynx, subcutaneous emphysema to face, neck, and upper chest.

Investigations
- CT may demonstrate laryngeal rupture with surgical emphysema.
- Plain X-ray or CT cervical spine.

Immediate management
- Urgent senior anaesthetic input to control airway if required.
- In the event of a complete airway obstruction and inability to intubate the patient, a surgical airway will be required.
- Urgent ENT review.
- Oxygen, monitoring, and IV access.
- Ensure in-line stabilization of cervical spine until injury excluded.

Pitfalls
Difficult intubation and airway control due to distorted anatomy.

☼ **Pulmonary contusion**

A pulmonary contusion is an injury to the lung parenchyma resulting in blood in the alveolar spaces, oedema, and loss of normal lung function.

Presentation
Mechanism and predisposing factors
- High energy blunt chest injury.
- Associated with rib fractures or flail chest.
- Common in children.
- Also found in blast injury with no external chest wall signs.

Signs, symptoms, and clinical findings
- Associated bruising to the chest wall, rib fractures, or flail chest.
- Mild hypomobility of the chest on the affected side.
- Non-specific crepitations or reduced air entry on auscultation.

Investigations
CXR
- Non-specific patchy opacification, sometimes difficult to differentiate from haemothorax or aspiration.
- Often lags 24–48 h behind the clinical picture.

CT scan
- Very sensitive in detecting pulmonary contusion.
- Can differentiate from atelectasis or aspiration.
- Contusions only detected on CT scan may not be clinically significant to cause respiratory problems.

Management
- **Supportive:** supplemental oxygen, analgesia, and chest physiotherapy. Maintain euvolaemia. Serial ABG's and close monitoring to detect any respiratory deterioration.
- RSI and mechanical ventilation for respiratory failure.

Complications
- ARDS.
- Respiratory failure.
- Atelectasis.
- Pneumonia.

:Ø: Cardiac contusion

Cardiac contusion is the most commonly missed fatal thoracic injury. The right ventricle is most commonly injured due to its position behind the sternum.

Presentation

Mechanism and predisposing factors
- Rapid deceleration injury.
- Direct compression or blow to the anterior chest wall.
- Sternal fracture.

Signs, symptoms, and clinical findings
- Chest pain.
- Cardiogenic shock.
- Arrythmias or conduction defects.

Investigations

ECG
Non-specific ST segment or T wave changes, multiple ventricular ectopics, unexplained sinus tachycardia, conduction defects, or RBBB.

Cardiac enzymes
Troponin I or Troponin T may be elevated, but can also be raised in hypo-volaemic shock or a non-significant cardiac injury.

Echo
TOE is more reliable than TTE to detect wall motion abnormalities, ventricular dysfunction, or pericardial effusion.

Management
- Cardiac monitoring.
- Early cardiology opinion.
- May rarely require anti-arrhythmic drugs or pacemaker insertion for conduction defects.
- Inotropes for cardiogenic shock.
- Associated coronary artery injury or injury to smaller vessels within the contused area may require surgical intervention.

Complications
- Arrhythmias.
- Ventricular dysfunction leading to cardiac failure.
- Pericardial effusion leading to tamponade.

Pitfalls
Remember traumatic injury may be the result of an acute medical emergency, e.g. cardiac arrhythmia or myocardial infarction, causing a collision. This may present in a similar manner.

☠ Traumatic aortic disruption

Aortic rupture is a common cause of sudden death following trauma and approximately 90% will be immediately fatal. The early survivors are likely to have an incomplete laceration with an intact adventitial layer and a contained haematoma. Survival of these patients relies on early diagnosis and urgent surgical repair.

The most common site of rupture is at the ligamentum arteriosum.

Presentation

Mechanism and predisposing factors

There are two theories of injury from rapid deceleration:

- Shearing between the mobile arch and the fixed descending thoracic aorta.
- The 'osseous pinch' theory with the first rib and clavicle swinging down to directly nip the aorta.

Signs, symptoms, and clinical findings

- Chest or back pain.
- Persistent or recurrent signs of hypovolaemic shock.
- Systolic murmur.
- Absent or reduced peripheral pulses. Asynchronous radial-radial or radial-femoral pulses. A different blood pressure between the arms and the arms and legs.

Investigations

CXR

Signs of aortic disruption (see Fig. 5.5) on plain CXR include:

- Widened mediastinum (>8 cm at level of aortic arch).
- Fractured first or second ribs.
- Pleural cap (apical haematoma).
- Depressed left main bronchus.
- Elevation and right shift of right main bronchus.
- Loss of definition of the aortic knuckle.
- Tracheal deviation to the right.
- Left haemothorax.
- Deviation of nasogastric tube in oesophagus to right.
- Obliteration of aortic window between pulmonary artery and aorta.

CT scan

Contrast CT can only be utilized if the patient is haemodynamically stable. If the CT scan is negative for mediastinal haematoma and aortic rupture, no further imaging is necessary. If the CT scan is positive with inadequate visualization of all vessels or the CT scan is equivocal, angiography is required.

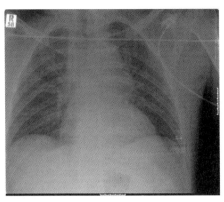

Fig. 5.5 Traumatic aortic disruption.

Management

• Discuss with the on-call Cardiothoracic team.
• Haemodynamically unstable patients require emergency operative intervention to control haemorrhage.
• Haemodynamically stable patients require control of blood pressure, avoidance of over aggressive fluid therapy and further imaging to define the extent of injury, until definitive repair (stenting or open repair).

Pitfalls

Beware the CXR may be normal despite the presence of aortic disruption. Equally, the mediastinum may look widened on a supine film in a normal patient. Obtain an urgent radiological opinion where any uncertainty exists.

:O: **Traumatic diaphragmatic injury**

Rupture of the diaphragm is uncommon following trauma. It is more likely to occur on the left side, as the right hemidiaphragm is relatively protected by the liver (Fig. 5.6). Right-sided ruptures are associated with a higher mortality due to severe associated injuries. Bilateral diaphragm ruptures are extremely rare.

Presentation

Mechanism and predisposing factors

- Blunt chest trauma, e.g. RTC, crush injury to abdomen causing a raised intra-abdominal pressure. This results in large radial tears with early herniation of abdominal viscera.
- Penetrating trauma, e.g. stab wounds, or GSW to chest or abdomen. This usually results in small diaphragmatic perforations, which gradually enlarge over days to weeks before herniation occurs.

Signs, symptoms, and clinical findings

- SOB, chest/abdominal pain, worse laying down.
- Reduced breath sounds on affected side, dull to percussion, presence of bowel sounds in chest.
- Hypoxia and respiratory failure from compression of lung on affected side.
- Haemodynamic instability if mediastinum compressed by herniated contents.
- Unexpected finding of abdominal contents in the thorax during thoracostomy for chest drain insertion.

Investigations

- **CXR:** elevation of hemi-diaphragm. Bowel, stomach, or NGT in chest; ipsilateral pleural effusion.
- **CT scan:** poorly visualizes diaphragm and, therefore, is not 100% sensitive at detecting injury.

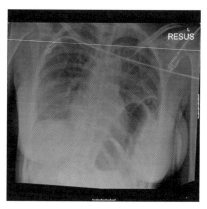

Fig. 5.6 Traumatic diaphragm rupture.

Immediate management

- Oxygen, IV access, IV analgesia.
- Insert nasogastric tube (NGT) to decompress gastric contents.
- ABG to establish if respiratory failure is present.
- ICU review as patient may require positive-pressure ventilation.
- Immediate senior surgical opinion. Patient may require either thoracoscopy, thoracotomy, or laparatomy for definitive assessment and direct repair.
- May require chest drain insertion on affected side to drain any associated haemo- or pneumothorax. This should be performed with great caution to avoid injury to herniated abdominal contents and only after senior review.

Complications

- Tension gastrothorax.
- Re-expansion pulmonary oedema.
- Infarction of bowel.
- Diaphragmatic paralysis.
- Empyema.

Pitfalls

Diaphragm rupture is a difficult diagnosis and often delayed. The CXR findings are often misinterpreted as an elevated hemi-diaphragm, acute gastric dilatation, or a loculated pneumo-haemothorax.

Insertion of a NGT followed by CXR may confirm the stomach is located in the hemithorax.

⚙ Oesophageal injury

Mechanism and predisposing factors
- Penetrating injury is most common.
- Blunt compression of upper abdomen or lower chest.

Signs, symptoms, and clinical findings
- Chest or back pain out of proportion to apparent injury.
- Subcutaneous emphysema in the neck.
- Haematemesis.
- Dysphagia.
- Signs of left pneumothorax or haemothorax.
- Particulate matter in any inserted chest tube.

Investigations
- CXR: pneumomediastinum, left pneumothorax, or pleural effusion.
- Contrast study and/or endoscopy for stable patients.

Immediate management
- Oxygen, monitoring, and IV access with X-match.
- Insertion of chest drain for any pneumothorax or haemothorax.
- IV antibiotics.
- Urgent surgical opinion.

Complications
- Mediastinitis and empyema.
- Long-term dysphagia and stricture formation.

☠ Mediastinal penetrating injury

Penetrating objects that traverse the mediastinum have the potential to injure the heart, great vessels, tracheobronchial tree, oesophagus, and lungs. Overall, the mortality is 20%.

Mechanism and predisposing factors

Stabbing, GSW, impalement on object, blast fragmentation.

Signs, symptoms, and clinical findings

- Entry and/or exit wounds.
- Signs of tension pneumothorax (see 📖 Tension pneumothorax, p60), open pneumothorax (see 📖 Open pneumothorax, p63), massive haemothorax (see 📖 Haemothorax, p64) or cardiac tamponade (see 📖 Cardiac tamponade, p68).

Investigations

- **CXR:** pneumothorax, foreign body, widened mediastinum.
- **FAST USS:** free fluid in pericardial sac.
- CT for stable patients, with contrast vascular and gastrointestinal (GI) studies.
- 12-lead ECG and echocardiogram (Echo) if suspected cardiac injury.

Immediate management

- Oxygen, monitoring, and IV access with X-match.
- Treat any life-threatening airway or chest injury.
- IV fluid boluses to maintain a SBP 90 mmHg.
- Remove all patients clothing (avoiding cutting through ballistic holes) and keep for police evidence.
- Search for wounds including a log roll to look at the back, and checking the groin, buttocks, perineum, and axilla.
- Seek urgent surgical opinion.
- Analgesia, e.g. titrated IV morphine.
- Treat wounds by cleaning, application of sterile dressing, check need for tetanus prophylaxis and IV antibiotics according to hospital policy.

Pitfalls

Under-estimating small external wounds, which have no correlation with the degree of internal injury.

⚠ Simple rib fractures

Mechanism and predisposing factors
Blunt trauma.

Signs, symptoms, and clinical findings
- Chest pain worse on inspiration and movement.
- Tenderness, swelling and crepitus overlying the fractures.
- Check for signs of flail chest (see 📖 Flail chest, p66).
- Check for signs of associated pneumothorax or haemothorax.

Investigations
No investigations are required unless there is clinical suspicion of under-lying lung injury, in which case CXR is indicated. 50% of rib fractures are not apparent on CXR.

Immediate management
- **Isolated rib fractures:** oral analgesia, e.g. co-codamol (paracetemol 1g QDS +/− opiate) diclofenac. Send home with general practitioner (GP) follow-up. Advise breathing exercises and to hold chest when coughing.
- **Multiple rib fractures:** treat like a flail chest. Intravenous analgesia, e.g. morphine. ABG to assess any respiratory inadequacy. Admission for analgesia and physiotherapy.

Complications
- Pneumonia.
- Pneumothorax.
- Respiratory failure.
- Haemothorax from intercostal vessel injury.

Who to send home
- Patients with isolated rib fracture.
- No pre-existing lung disease.
- Young patient with no pre-existing morbidities.
- Adequate inspiratory effort after oral analgesia.
- No other lung injuries identified after full assessment.

Pitfalls
Under-estimating the extent of a chest wall injury and consequences of rib fractures on patient's respiratory function.

⚙ Sternal fracture

Presentation
Mechanism and predisposing factors
- Seat belt or steering wheel impact in RTC's.
- Direct blow to chest, e.g. kicked by horse.

Signs, symptoms, and clinical findings
- Anterior chest pain.
- Localized swelling and tenderness over sternum.

Investigations
ECG & cardiac enzymes
To exclude cardiac contusion (see 📖 Cardiac contusion, p75).

CXR and lateral sternal X-ray
To demonstrate any sternal fracture or associated lung injury.

Management
- Cardiac monitor, supplementary oxygen.
- Adequate analgesia.

Who to send home
Isolated sternal fractures in young patients with no pre-existing lung disease, with no other traumatic injury, with normal ECG and cardiac markers, and whose pain can be adequately controlled with oral analgesia may be safe for discharge.

Complications
- Cardiac contusion.
- Pulmonary contusion.
- Great vessel injury.
- Chest infection (late).

Pitfalls
Beware that sternal fractures resulting from high-energy transfer may be associated with upper thoracic fractures.

Abdominal trauma

☠ Assessment of abdominal injury

The abdomen is one of the five sites of life-threatening haemorrhage in the trauma patient and should be assessed as part of the circulatory assessment in the primary survey.

The boundaries of the abdomen are from the nipples at full expiration to the inguinal ligaments and pubic symphysis anteriorly, and the tips of the scapula to the gluteal skin crease posteriorly. Remember that lower chest trauma may cause abdominal injury.

The abdomen is divided into the:
- Peritoneal cavity (including liver, spleen, stomach, parts of duodenum and bowel).
- The retroperitoneum (including major vessels, kidneys, ureters, colon).
- The pelvic cavity (including bladder, rectum, iliac vessels, and internal genitalia in females).

Diagnosis of an abdominal injury is very difficult particularly in a multiple injury patient who may have reduced conscious level or distracting injury. Missed injury is associated with a poor outcome.

Presentation

Mechanism of injury
- Blunt (see 📖 Blunt abdominal trauma, p90).
- Penetrating (see 📖 Penetrating abdominal trauma, p92).
- Blast injury (see 📖 Blast injury, p91).

It is important to take a detailed history from the patient, paramedic, or police regarding the mechanism of injury to assess the likelihood of abdominal injury.

Signs, symptoms, and clinical findings
- Abdominal pain.
- Inspection:
  - pattern bruising, e.g. seat belt sign;
  - wounds to anterior or posterior abdomen;
  - distension (late sign).
- Abdominal tenderness on palpation or peritonism.
- Auscultation for bowel sounds (may be difficult in Resuscitation room and not a reliable sign).
- Rectal or vaginal bleeding – PR for rectal integrity and tone.
- Tachycardia and/or hypotension.

Beware significant amounts of blood may be present in the abdominal cavity without any clinical signs.

Investigations

- **Bloods:** may be normal despite significant injury.
- **Plain abdominal X-ray:** is rarely useful and an erect CXR to assess for free gas is generally not possible in a trauma patient.
- **Urinalysis:** for blood on dipstick and a pregnancy test in all women of child-bearing age. A catheter may be required to obtain a urine sample.
- FAST USS (see 📖 Investigation of abdominal injury, p88).
- CT scan (see 📖 Investigation of abdominal injury, p88).

Initial management of abdominal injury

- Treat airway and breathing problems.
- Oxygen 15 L.
- Insert 2 × wide bore IV access.
- Send bloods for FBC, U&E, LFT, amylase, clotting and X match.
- Give IV sodium chloride 0.9% in 250 mL boluses to maintain SBP above 90 mmHg.
- Involve a surgeon at an early stage.
- Inform the duty anaesthetist and theatres if the patient is likely to require an early laparotomy.
- Consider the need for a NGT to decompress the stomach and reduce risk of vomiting.
- Insert a urinary catheter and monitor hourly urine output. This should not be performed before urological input if there are any signs of urethral injury, e.g. blood at meatus, scrotal, or perineal haematoma, significant pelvic fracture and patient unable to self-void.

Pitfalls

Log-rolling a patient with intra-abdominal injury may lead to disruption of clots and catastrophic internal haemorrhage with shock. Try to minimize movements using a scoop stretcher or pat slide.

A compromise may have to be met to thoroughly assess the back and flanks for posterior abdominal injury and rectal examination. Depending on the mechanism of injury, this may include a gloved hand passed under the patient to check for bleeding or wounds, or a limited 15° log roll each side to directly visualize the back.

⑦ Investigation of abdominal injury

Focused assessment with sonography for trauma ultrasound scan

FAST is used for the rapid assessment of free fluid in the abdominal cavity or the pericardium as an adjunct to the primary survey.

Advantages
- Rapid, non-invasive bedside test.
- Can be performed in the Resuscitation room by a trained emergency medicine or surgical doctor on haemodynamically unstable patients.
- Easily repeated.

Disadvantages
- Requires approximately 500 mL blood to have accumulated before reliable detection.
- A negative test does not exclude intra-abdominal haemorrhage.
- Operator dependent.
- Views limited by surgical emphysema, bowel gas, or obesity.
- Does not identify which organ is injured or the type of fluid, e.g. blood or bowel contents.

FAST assesses the presence of free fluid (black) in four areas:
- Hepatorenal recess in right upper quadrant (between liver and right kidney).
- Splenorenal recess in left upper quadrant (between spleen and left kidney).
- Pouch of Douglas in pelvis (behind the bladder).
- Pericardium (around the heart).

If haemodynamically unstable patient
- **FAST positive:** needs laparotomy.
- **FAST negative:** look for other sources of haemorrhage.

If haemodynamically stable patient
- **FAST positive:** needs CT to define injury.
- **FAST negative:** repeat scan in 20–30 min.

Diagnostic peritoneal lavage

This used to be the investigation of choice for identifying abdominal injury in unstable patients in the Resuscitation room or where other radiological investigations were not available. It has been superseded in most centres by use of FAST ultrasound and the availability of CT scans. The test is invasive, with risk of iatrogenic damage to abdominal organs, and there is a high rate of false positive tests.

Prior to diagnostic peritoneal lavage (DPL) the bladder is decompressed with a urinary catheter and the stomach with a NGT. The procedure involves cleaning the skin and injecting local anaesthetic at the site of puncture midline just below the umbilicus. The skin is elevated with forceps, and incised down to fascia and then through peritoneum. A peritoneal dialysis catheter is inserted into the peritoneal cavity and aspirated.

If this is negative, 1 L of warmed sodium chloride 0.9% is instilled via the catheter, agitated, and then re-aspirated. A sample of the fluid is sent to the laboratory.

A positive scan is free aspiration of >10 mL of blood, gastrointestinal contents or bile, or on lavage >100,000 red blood cells (RBC), >500 white blood cells (WBC) or a positive Gram stain test. A negative test does not exclude retroperitoneal injury or diaphragmatic tears.

CT scan

CT scan may be performed as part of a total body CT scan in the multiple-injured patient or to specifically evaluate abdominal injuries. Intravenous contrast is used, and the scan includes the top of diaphragm (to identify haemothorax or pneumothorax) down to the pubic symphysis and pelvis.

The advantage of CT is visualization of retroperitoneal structures, detection of arterial contrast extravasation and the ability to grade solid organ injury, which may allow non-operative management. It may miss some diaphragmatic, hollow viscus, or early pancreas injuries.

Disadvantages include exposure to ionizing radiation and side effects of intravenous contrast. The main limitation of CT is it cannot be used in haemodynamically unstable patients. However, in experienced trauma centres with modern high-speed CT scanners situated in proximity to the Resuscitation room and a specialized senior team accompanying the patient, transient responders to resuscitation may also be scanned. This decision must be made by a senior experienced Trauma team leader.

Interventional radiology

Angiography may be useful to accurately diagnose bleeding sites and therapeutically embolize vessels. This is particularly useful following complex pelvic fractures and in solid organ injury with vascular damage.

Summary

Haemodynamically UNSTABLE + clinical signs of intra-abdominal bleeding = laparotomy

Haemodynamically UNSTABLE + uncertainty if any intra-abdominal bleeding = FAST USS (or DPL)

Haemodynamically STABLE with clinical signs or uncertainty = CT scan (as may be managed non-operatively)

:☹: **Blunt abdominal trauma**

This is the commonest cause of abdominal trauma in the UK. The most commonly injured organs are the liver and spleen.

Mechanism
- RTC.
- Crush injury, e.g. industrial.
- Fall from height.
- Direct blow, e.g. punch, kick from horse.

Pattern of injury
- Direct impact causing compression or crush injury.
- Deceleration, shearing and rotational forces.
- Increased intra-luminal pressure causing injury to hollow viscus.

Important features in history
Speed of vehicle, site of impact, use of seat belt, air bag deployment, vehicle intrusion, position of patient in vehicle after impact, entrapment of torso.

Indications for further investigation
- Mechanism of injury gives high index of suspicion.
- Injuries above and below abdomen, e.g. chest and femurs.
- Clinical signs including bruising.
- Difficult to assess for abdominal injury, e.g. reduced conscious level, distracting injury, spinal injury.
- Lower rib fractures may suggest liver or splenic injury.

Non-operative management
This may be an option for certain isolated blunt liver, spleen, or renal injuries. The decision must be made by a senior surgeon with awareness that the patient may deteriorate and require surgical intervention later. The indications are:
- Injuries to solid organs demonstrated by CT to be appropriate for non-operative management.
- Minimal physical signs.
- Haemodynamically stable (<2 units of blood transfused).
- HDU/ICU bed available to observe patient.
- Senior surgeon available to perform repeated serial examinations and perform urgent laparotomy if later required.

Indications for laparotomy
- Haemodynamically unstable with positive clinical signs.
- Haemodynamically unstable with positive FAST scan.
- Haemodynamically stable with positive CT scan (unsuitable for non-operative management).

☼ Blast injury

Explosions from domestic gas, industrial sites, or bombs may cause abdominal injury by:

- **Primary blast wave:** causing perforation of bowel or shearing of mesentery or solid organs (without any external signs of injury).
- **Secondary fragmentation injury:** penetration of abdominal cavity by bomb materials or flying debris.
- **Tertiary blunt injury:** from being thrown by the blast wind.

Signs and symptoms of primary blast injury
- Abdominal pain, nausea and vomiting, tenesmus, testicular pain.
- Abdominal distension and tenderness.
- Rectal bleeding.
- Tachycardia and hypotension.

Injuries from primary blast injury
- Intestinal haemorrhage.
- Intestinal perforation.
- Mesenteric tears.
- Solid organ rupture (liver, spleen, kidney, or diaphragm).
- Retroperitoneal haemorrhage.

Management
- Assess and treat any life-threatening airway or chest injury.
- Manage as blunt or penetrating abdominal injury according to findings.
- Admit for observation if there are no obvious features of abdominal injury on examination or investigation, as there is a high risk of delayed intestinal perforation (up to 10 days).
- Low threshold for laparotomy.

☠ Penetrating abdominal injury

Stab wounds are still more common than GSW in the UK. Injuries depend on the energy transferred by the penetrating object and the trajectory.

Mechanism
- Stabbing.
- GSW.
- Fragmentation in explosion.
- Impalement.

Assessment
- A full history should include the time of injury, type of weapon or round, distance from assailant, number of wounds or shots, position of patient when penetration occurred, and the amount of external bleeding at scene.
- It is essential to fully expose the patient early in the primary survey to identify any concealed wounds. This includes the back, flanks, groins, buttocks, and perineum plus a rectal examination.
- **Beware: the size of the external wound does not determine the likelihood or severity of intra-abdominal injuries.**
- In a conscious patient check for a spinal cord injury by assessing the neurological status of the limbs.
- Plain X-ray may be useful in stable patients to identify the location of any retained bullet and allow prediction of the trajectory, e.g. has it gone from chest to thigh, passing through the thorax and abdominal cavity?

Foreign bodies
Any foreign body or knife must only be removed in theatre at laparotomy under direct vision to enable control of any potential haemorrhage or contamination.

Wound care
- Cover wound with sterile dressing. Any protruding bowel or omentum should be covered with warm saline soaked swabs, and not handled or pushed back into the abdomen.
- Check tetanus status and consider need for prophylaxis.
- Give IV antibiotics according to local prescribing guidelines.

Additional investigations in penetrating trauma
Local wound exploration
Local wound exploration is the evaluation of a stab wound using local anaesthetic before extending and probing the wound. This should only be performed in theatre by a surgeon who will be able to proceed to laparoscopy or laparotomy if it is indicated. Exploration is positive when the anterior fasica or peritoneum has been breached. There is no role for wound exploration in GSW: these should all have a laparotomy.

Serial examinations
Serial examination has good sensitivity and negative predictive value for evaluating patients with minor penetrating abdominal trauma. The patient is admitted for observation for at least 24 h with hourly assessment of haemodynamic status and at least 4-hourly assessment for clinical abdominal signs. If the patient develops any signs of bleeding or peritonism during this period of observation a laparotomy is performed. If they develop a pyrexia, tachycardia, or localized tenderness a CT scan, laparoscopy, or laparotomy is performed. If after 24 h, the patient remains well they can start a normal diet and discharge can be considered.

Laparoscopy
Diagnostic laparoscopy (under general anaesthetic in theatre) may be useful for identifying peritoneal penetration following abdominal stab wounds or diaphragmatic injury. It may miss a bowel injury or retroperitoneal injury.

Indications for laparotomy
- Stab wounds with peritoneal penetration.
- Any GSW to the abdomen.
- Evisceration.
- Retained foreign bodies.
- Peritonitis.
- Haemodynamically unstable with penetrating abdominal injury.
- Haemodynamically stable with positive CT scan.

Pitfalls
Missing penetrating injury to the buttocks, groin, or back with abdominal or rectal injury.

Forensics
Ensure a member of staff informs the police that you have 'a patient' in the department with a stab wound or GSW. If the patient has arrived by the ambulance service they will usually be accompanied by a police officer. It is justifiable to break confidentiality when there are issues of public interest, and to protect the safety of your department and staff. Consult the General Medical Council website and the MPS/MDU for further information.

Ensure all the patients clothes, belongings, and any weapons are kept secure to be given to an identified police officer for forensic examination.

Head injury

☠ Head injury

Head injury is present in 50% of trauma deaths. There are over 1 million Emergency department attendances per year, of which 90% are minor head injuries.

Primary brain injury is the result of the mechanical events that occur at the time of the injury and can only be influenced by prevention, e.g. cycle helmets, seatbelts, vehicle air bags, etc.

Secondary brain injury is the subsequent neurological damage caused by hypoxia, hypo or hypercapnia, hypovolaemia, oedema causing raised ICP, seizures, or later infections.

Many head injuries will be associated with alcohol or drug intoxication. However, the clinician must never assume a deterioration of conscious level or agitation is due to intoxication, rather than the effects of a head injury.

Presentation

Mechanism and predisposing factors

- **Blunt:** RTC, assault, fall from height, sporting events, e.g. horse riding.
- **Penetrating (rare):** stab, GSW, impalement.

Important facts in history

- Mechanism of injury?
- Any medical cause for the head injury and unresponsiveness, e.g. hypoglycaemia, epileptic seizure?
- Any witnessed loss of consciousness?
- Any amnesia of events before (retrograde) or after (anterograde) injury?
- Any vomiting?
- Any headache?
- Any abnormal drowsiness, blurred vision, or fits?
- What was the GCS when the ambulance arrived?
- Any PMH of epilepsy or clotting disorders?
- Are they taking warfarin or another anticoagulant?
- Any drug or alcohol ingestion?
- Who is at home with them normally?

Physiology

Monro-Kellie doctrine

The intracranial contents consist of brain, venous blood, arterial blood, and cerebrospinal fluid contained within a rigid container of the skull. When a mass develops inside the skull (e.g. bleed or swelling) venous blood and CSF are extruded to keep the intracranial pressure (ICP) normal at 5–10 mmHg.

A point comes when no further compensation is possible and the ICP increases massively.

If unrelieved, coning will occur, with herniation of the temporal lobe causing an ipsilateral third nerve palsy and contralateral hemiparesis, and a Cushing's response with bradypnoea, bradycardia, and hypertension.

Autoregulation with blood pressure

Cerebral blood flow is kept constant by the cerebral arterioles responding to the blood pressure – constricting in response to low pressure and dilating in response to high pressure.

However, following a head injury this autoregulation is disturbed so that cerebral blood flow is dependent on cerebral perfusion pressure (CPP).

CPP = Mean arterial pressure – Intracranial pressure

Therefore, in the presence of an elevated ICP is it imperative to maintain the mean arterial blood pressure (MAP) to ensure adequate CPP.

Carbon dioxide

- Hypocapnia causes cerebral arterioles to constrict with a reduction in cerebral blood flow.
- Hypercapnia causes cerebral arterioles to vasodilate, resulting in an increased volume in the cranium and, therefore, a raised ICP.
- The aim is to achieve normocapnia.

⑦ Assessment of head injury

Primary survey

The initial assessment of the head-injured patient is the same as any other trauma patient – assessing ABC to exclude any other injury including:

- High suspicion of cervical spine injury with full immobilization.
- Examination for bleeding scalp wounds as part of circulation remembering concealed occipital haemorrhage.

Disability assessment should include:

- AVPU score initially.

Then:

- GCS score recorded as E-V-M.
- Pupils for size, symmetry, and reaction to light (remember direct trauma to the eye may cause a mydriasis with pupil dilatation on the affected side).
- Limb power.
- Bedside blood glucose.

Secondary survey

Examination for signs of facial fracture

Bruising, swelling, deformity, bony tenderness, diplopia or an inability to perform eye movements, paraesthesia over skin, epistaxis.

Examination for signs of basal skull fracture

- Bilateral peri-orbital bruising.
- Rhinnorhea or ottorhea (indicates an open fracture).
- Haemotympanum or bleeding from auditory meatus.
- Subconjunctival haemorrhage with no posterior margin seen.
- Battles sign – bruising over the mastoid process without any direct trauma to this area (normally develops >24 h after injury).

Examination of scalp

- Any wounds, bleeding, swelling, or foreign body?
- A log roll may need to be performed to visualize all of the scalp.

Full neurological examination

Including cranial nerves and peripheral nervous system in the co-operative patient.

AVPU score

- Is the patient **A**lert?
- Do they respond to **V**oice?
- Do they only respond to **P**ain?
- Are they **U**nresponsive?

Glasgow Coma Score

Eye opening
Spontaneous   4
To voice   3
To pain   2
None   1

Best verbal response
Orientated   5
Confused   4
Inappropriate words   3
Incomprehensible sounds   2
None   1

Best motor response
The most accurate indicator of prognosis
Obeys commands   6
Localizes painful stimulus   5
Withdraws from painful stimulus   4
Abnormal flexion (decerebrate)   3
Abnormal extension (decorticate)   2
None   1

GCS should be recorded according to each response, e.g. GCS 10 = E3 V2 M5.

Paediatric GCS for under 5 years

Best verbal response
Alert, babbles, words to usual ability   5
Less than usual, irritable cry   4
Cries to pain   3
Moans to pain   2
None   1

Also 'normal spontaneous movements' instead of 'obeys commands' for motor score of 6.

⑦ Imaging of head injury

Skull X-rays

Skull X-rays have been largely superseded by CT scan. The only indications now are suspected foreign body in minor head injury, e.g. glass to scalp wound or suspected non-accidental injury (NAI) in children (requested by senior paediatrician).

CT scan

NICE head injury guidelines (2007) recommend that a CT scan should be performed within 1 h if there is:
- GCS <13 on initial assessment in the Emergency department.
- GCS <15 at 2 h after injury.
- Suspected open or depressed skull fracture.
- Clinical signs of basal skull fracture.
- More than one episode of vomiting.
- Post-traumatic seizure (not known epileptic).
- Focal neurological deficit.

A CT scan should be performed within 8 h if:
- There has been loss of consciousness (LOC) or amnesia >30 min before impact.
AND:
- The patient is age >65 years.
- OR has a coagulopathy (including current treatment with warfarin).
- OR dangerous mechanism of injury:
  - e.g. pedestrian or cyclist struck by a motor vehicle;
  - occupant ejected from a motor vehicle;
  - fall from >1 m or >5 stairs.

For children (<16 years) an immediate CT scan should be requested for:
- Witnessed LOC > 5 min or amnesia > 5 min.
- Abnormal drowsiness.
- Three or more discrete episodes of vomiting.
- Clinical suspicion of non-accidental injury.
- GCS <14 on initial assessment (GCS <15 if infant under 1 year).
- Suspicion of open or depressed skull fracture.
- Any sign of basal skull fracture.
- Focal neurological deficit.
- Dangerous mechanism of injury, e.g. RTC >40 mph, fall from height >3 m, high speed injury from projectile or object.
- Infants with bruise/swelling/laceration of more than 5 cm on head.

Types of head injury

Skull fractures

The presence of a skull fracture increases the likelihood of intracranial pathology. These patients should have a CT head and be admitted for observation.

Contusions

Contusions on a CT scan require admission for observation as they may form an intracranial bleed or cause cerebral oedema requiring neurosurgical intervention.

Diffuse brain injury

Range from mild concussion to persistent coma. The CT will initially appear normal or have diffuse oedema with loss of the normal grey-white distinction of brain matter. MRI is better at detecting diffuse axonal injury.

Extradural (epidural) bleed

The bleed is located between the skull and the dura, and is biconvex in shape on a CT scan. It is commonly caused by a temporal fracture producing a tear in the middle meningeal artery. After the head injury there may be a lucid interval before deterioration in the conscious level. Extradural bleeds carry a good prognosis if evacuated as they are associated with little brain substance injury.

Subdural bleed

The bleed is located between the dura and arachnoid mater, and is concave covering the surface of the hemisphere on CT scan. Subdurals are often associated with tearing of bridging veins of the cerebral cortex and, therefore, are more common in alcoholics or the elderly who have atrophic brains with a larger space.

There is a poorer prognosis as they are frequently associated with underlying brain damage.

Traumatic subarachnoid haemorrhage

Bleeding into the subarachnoid space and ventricles is a common accompanying feature of major head trauma. If significant in volume, it is usually associated with a poor outcome.

☠ Management of head injury

Airway

Involve the anaesthetist immediately for any patient with GCS <15. Early RSI and intubation will be necessary for the following patients:

- GCS ≤8.
- Loss of protective laryngeal reflexes and vomiting.
- Ventilatory insufficiency:
  - hypoxaemia (PaO_2 < 13 kPa on oxygen);
  - hypercarbia ($PaCO_2$ > 6 kPa).
- Significantly deteriorating conscious level (1 or more points on motor score), even if not coma.
- Unstable fractures of the facial skeleton.
- Copious bleeding into mouth.
- Seizures.

❶ Check GCS, motor power, and pupils prior to induction, and paralysis agents.

❶ Remember, induction agents may cause hypotension and laryngoscopy may cause a raised ICP.

Intubation is often difficult due to:

- Manual in-line stabilization preventing optimal positioning for intubation.
- Facial trauma.
- High risk of regurgitation and aspiration.

Cervical spine

- Ensure the cervical spine is fully immobilized until an injury has been clinically and radiologically excluded.

❶ Beware cervical collars may increase ICP by up to 4 mmHg if they are applied too tight.

Breathing

- Identify and manage any life-threatening chest injuries.
- Early oxygen.
- Aim for PaO_2 >13 kPa and $PaCO_2$ 4.5 kPa.
- Provide ventilation at appropriate rate if patients spontaneous respiration is inadequate.

Circulation

- Identify and manage any external or internal haemorrhage. FAST scan the abdomen to exclude any intra-abdominal bleed, and obtain portable chest and pelvic X-rays to exclude other sources of non-compressible haemorrhage.
- Scalp wounds may bleed profusely and require immediate suturing to control haemorrhage. These emergency sutures can be removed and replaced with cosmetically appropriate sutures once the patient is stable.
- Maintain a MAP ~100 mmHg by giving fluid boluses and inotropes if required. Remember CPP = MAP – ICP. Hypotension doubles the mortality from a severe head injury. This may cause conflict with principles of hypotensive resuscitation in non-compressible haemorrhage, e.g. intra-abdominal bleed, but without adequate blood pressure there will be no cerebral perfusion.
- Send bloods, including clotting. If the patient is on warfarin with a suspected intracranial haemorrhage and neurological signs, the raised INR can be reversed by giving vitamin K 10 mg IV and fresh frozen plasma (FFP). Liase with the local haematologist for advice.

Disability

- Check bedside blood glucose and maintain normoglycaemia. This includes using an insulin sliding scale or infusion if the patient is diabetic with grossly abnormal levels.
- Seizures may complicate a head injury. Maintain airway and ensure the patient is receiving oxygen. Call anaesthetist immediately. Give IV lorazepam 4 mg or IV Diazemuls® 10 mg. Give a second dose if the patient is still fitting after 10 min. If the patient is not normally on antiepileptic drugs, load with phenytoin 18 mg/kg, diluted in 100 mL sodium chloride 0.9% over 30 min.
- Mannitol 20% (0.5 g/kg) is an osmotic diuretic, which may be needed to reduce ICP prior to definitive neurosurgery. It should only be used on the advice of a neurosurgeon.
- Steroids have no role. A multicentre randomized control trial in 2004 found higher mortality in head-injured patients treated with steroids vs. placebo.

⑦ Follow-up of head injury

Discuss with neurosurgeon
- Abnormal CT.
- Persisting coma (GCS ‚8) after initial resuscitation.
- Unexplained confusion for more than 4 h.
- Deterioration in GCS after admission (pay greater attention to motor response deterioration).
- Progressive focal neurological signs.
- Seizure without full recovery.
- Definite or suspected penetrating injury.
- CSF leak.
- Depressed skull fracture.

Minor head injury
Patients can be discharged from hospital if the following apply:
- GCS 15 or normal for patient (e.g. dementia patients).
- No continuing worrying signs, e.g. persistent vomiting or severe headache despite analgesia.
- No other injuries requiring admission.
- If CT was indicated, imaging is reported as normal.
- Competent supervision by adult at home.
- Carer capable of understanding verbal and written head injury advice.

Provide a prescription or advice on adequate analgesia, paracetemol +/− oral opiate (e.g. co-codamol) and ibuprofen. The patient should rest and not drink any alcohol for at least 24 h. If the patient has undergone CT imaging, give a letter for the GP with details of the clinical history, examination, and investigation results. Advise the patient to return to the Emergency department if there are any symptoms or signs that are of concern.

Special circumstances

☠ Cardiac arrest in trauma

Cardiac arrest following trauma carries an extremely poor prognosis. There are many irreversible causes, e.g. injury to the vital mediastinal structures, severe head injury, major tracheobronchial injury, or a medical cause of cardiac arrest leading up the traumatic event.

Basic and advanced life support (following the most recent Resuscitation Council guidelines) should be commenced immediately (see Fig. 8.1). The aim is to identify and manage any reversible causes early, to have the greatest chance of success.

The most common reversible causes in a trauma patient (in the 4 H's and 4 T's) will be:
- Airway obstruction leading to hypoxia.
- Tension Pneumothorax.
- Hypovolaemia.
- Cardiac tamponade.

Management

- Confirm cardiac arrest and start CPR 30:2
- **Airway:**
  - avoid head tilt–chin lift in the trauma patient;
  - ensure early intubation by a trained physician;
  - maintain cervical spine immobilization.
- **Breathing:**
  - ventilate with 15 L O_2;
  - perform bilateral open thoracostomies to exclude tension pneumothorax.
- **Circulation:**
  - control external haemorrhage;
  - wide bore IV access and 2 L crystalloid stat;
  - in the case of penetrating trauma to the chest or abdomen consider immediate emergency thoracotomy if time of arrest <10 min ago (**see** 📖 Emergency department thoracotomy, p50).
- **Disability:** check a bedside blood glucose.
- **Exposure:** remove patients clothing and make a rapid assessment of the extent of injury, e.g. if massive head injury with exposed brain tissue further resuscitation will be futile.

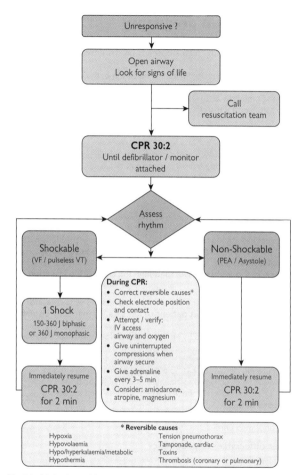

Fig. 8.1 Adult advanced life support algorithm. Reproduced with permission of The Resuscitation Council UK.

☠ Trauma in pregnancy

Trauma is the most common cause of non-obstetric death in pregnant women. Survival of the foetus depends on the effective resuscitation of the mother.

The gestational age is estimated by palpation of the uterus:
- Just out of the pelvis at 12 weeks.
- To the umbilicus at 20–22 weeks.
- Up to the costal margin by 34–36 weeks.

Changes in anatomy and physiology in pregnancy

Airway
- Increased risk of airway obstruction in the supine position and **difficulty intubating** from increased soft tissue.
- **High risk of aspiration** due to reduced gastrointestinal motility and competence of the oesophageal sphincter.

Breathing
- Increased oxygen consumption in pregnancy. ∴**Give high flow oxygen early**.
- Rise in tidal volume by 40% and physiological hyperventilation giving a normal $PaCO_2$ of around 4 kPa. ∴**Interpret ABG accordingly**.
- Diaphragm rises up to 4 cm as the uterus enlarges, so ensure any **thoracostomies are performed high for chest drain insertion**.

Circulation
- In the supine position, the uterus will compress the vena cava and cause hypotension. ∴**Tilt patient to left side, or manually displace uterus to left**.
- Blood volume increases by up to 40%. Therefore major haemorrhage of >1.5L can occur without signs of hypovolaemic shock. ∴**Consider fluids or blood earlier.**
- The uterine circulation has no autoregulation, therefore blood flow will be directly proportional to maternal blood pressure and any vasoconstriction in shock will compromise foetus. ∴**Avoid hypotension**.
- The uterus displaces abdominal organs making physical examination of the abdomen unreliable.

Other differences in pregnancy

Prescribing in pregnancy
Consult the British National Formulary (BNF) to check that drugs you are prescribing (analgesics, antibiotics, etc) are safe in pregnancy. For example, opiates cause respiratory depression in neonates and NSAIDs are contraindicated in the third trimester of pregnancy. Pregnant women also require lower doses of anaesthetic drugs.

Radiation exposure

Excessive radiation exposure can put the foetus at risk of teratogenesis, growth retardation, and childhood cancers. However X-rays on severely injured pregnant women should not be withheld in life-threatening circumstances. The risks are highest in the first trimester. Where possible use the lowest exposure, e.g. USS rather than CT, and use abdominal lead aprons during X-rays. Seek senior help to weigh up the risks and benefits, and liaise with the consultant radiologist on-call.

Rhesus group

Trauma can cause transplacental haemorrhage of foetal blood into the maternal circulation. A rhesus negative woman would then form antibodies to any foetal rhesus positive blood cells passing into the circulation. This would mount a reaction and cause potentially fatal haemolytic disease of the newborn.

For any sensitizing episode, e.g. trauma, check the rhesus blood group of the mother and perform a Kleihauer test, which will detect foetal red blood cells in the maternal circulation.

If the woman is rhesus negative, she will require anti-D immunoglobulin within 72 h. The dose is 250 units for <20 weeks gestation and 500 units for >20 weeks gestation. Seek advice from a senior in Obstetrics and Gynaecology.

Domestic violence

Violence by an intimate partner or family member is more common than we think, and the risk is greater for a woman when pregnant. Domestic violence often begins or escalates during pregnancy. Consider the diagnosis in any patient with the following:

- The explanation of mechanism of injury is not consistent with clinical findings.
- Delayed presentation.
- Partner insists on staying with patient for whole consultation and answer questions for them.
- Injuries to breasts, abdomen, or genitals.
- Repeated attendances to emergency department.
- Poor eye contact and self-blame by patient.

Offer the patient support, give them information regarding local domestic violence organizations, and encourage them to report to the police.

Management of the pregnant trauma patient

Call for Obstetric and Gynaecology Registrar or Consultant as soon as receive trauma alert or patient arrives in the department

ABC
See differences in anatomy and physiology.

Left lateral position if there is a visible 'bump'
- Patient strapped fully on a spinal board – tilt with blankets under the right side of the board.
- Patient on a trolley – displace uterus manually to the left with two hands. Once any life-threatening injuries and the spine have been cleared, the patient can be rolled onto her left side or tilted to the left with a wedge under the right hip.

Assessment of the foetus
History
- Obstetric history, any previous preterm labours or abruptions.
- Last menstrual period and expected date of delivery.
- Any abdominal pain, contractions, PV loss of blood, or clear fluid?
- Any foetal movements?

Examination
- Measure fundal height to predict gestational age.
- Look for uterine tenderness or rigidity, easily palpable foetal parts, external inspection for per vaginam (PV) bleeding or amniotic fluid loss.
- **Do not perform a PV examination.**
- Doppler USS for foetal heart rate.
- Look for pregnancy record 'green book', which mother normally carries with her at all times.
- Ask obstetrics and gynaecology (O&G) to assess patient early – abdomen, PV, cardiotocography (CTG), etc.

Specific injuries
Blunt injury
The bony pelvis, uterine wall and amniotic fluid act as protection for the foetus from blunt injury. A direct impact to the abdomen, compression by seatbelt in RTC, or deceleration shearing forces may cause uterine rupture or placental abruption.

Placental abruption
- This is the most common cause of foetal death after blunt trauma.
- **Symptoms and signs:** PV bleeding, uterine tenderness and rigidity, contractions, larger fundal height than expected for dates, hypovolaemic shock.
- **Treatment:** emergency Caesarean section.

Uterine rupture
- **Symptoms and signs:** PV bleeding, abdominal tenderness, loss of foetal movements, palpable extra-uterine foetal parts, hypovolaemic shock
- **Treatment:** emergency laparatomy, Caesarean section +/– hysterectomy.

Penetrating injury
A larger uterus protects the abdominal viscera from penetrating injury, but means a poor prognosis for the foetus if the uterus is penetrated.

Uterine penetration
- **Signs and symptoms:** penetrating wound to abdomen, loss of foetal movements, loss of foetal heart sounds, or bradycardia.
- **Treatment:** emergency laparatomy, Caesarean section.

Cardiac arrest in pregnancy
- Perimortem Caesarean section should be performed within 5 min of cardiac arrest if the uterine fundus is above the umbilicus or known gestation >24 weeks. Call for Obstetric and Paediatric support immediately.

☠ Trauma in children

Trauma is the leading cause of death in children. Their smaller size will influence the pattern and severity of injury, e.g. point of impact of a car bumper is higher on the body than an adult.

A structured ABCDE approach should be used in the same order of priority as for adults.

Differences in paediatric trauma patients

The size of a child and, therefore, equipment and drug doses vary with age. Use the child's age (look at the label in their clothing if you do not have a history) to calculate an estimated weight. Alternatively, use a Broselow tape if one is available.

$$\text{Weight in kg} = 2 \,(\text{age} + 4)$$

Airway
- Large tongue, small mouth = difficult intubation.
- Higher and more anterior larynx, therefore, easier to intubate with a straight blade laryngoscope.
- Carinal angles are symmetrical so it is possible to misplace endotracheal tube (ETT) down either bronchus.
- More prone to vomiting after insult.
- Size NPA diameter = child's nostril; length = nostril to tragus of ear.
- Size OPA as for adults, insert right way up with tongue depressor.
- Use an uncuffed ETT in smaller pre-pubertal children.
- Avoid surgical cricothyroidotomy in infants or young children – use needle cricothyroidotomy.

$$\text{Internal diameter of ETT} = \text{age}/4 + 4$$
$$\text{Length of oral ETT} = \text{age}/2 + 12$$

C spine
- Head is large, tending to cause neck flexion = cervical spine immobilization requires padding under the child's torso and shoulders to maintain neutral alignment.
- Spinal cord injury is very rare.
- Spinal cord injury without radiographic abnormalities (SCIWORA) is based on a history or examination of neurological deficit.

Breathing
Compliant ribs mean that serious underlying lung injury can occur without rib fractures. Rib fractures indicated severe force. Higher incidence of pulmonary contusions. See Table 8.1 for normal respiratory rate for different ages.

Table 8.1 Respiratory rates of children

Age in years	Respiratory rate
<1	30–40
1–2	25–35
2–5	20–30
5–12	20–25
>12	15–20

Circulation
- The overall circulating volume of blood is less than an adult, so small amounts of haemorrhage are significant.
- Children compensate well for hypovolaemia and then suddenly deteriorate. Hypotension is a pre-terminal sign.
- Liver and spleen injuries are common in children and often treated conservatively with observation.

See Table 8.2 for pulse and systolic blood pressure in children.

Table 8.2 Pulse and systolic BP in children

Age in years	Pulse	Systolic BP
<1	110–160	70–90
1–2	100–150	80–95
2–5	95–140	80–100
5–12	80–120	90–110
>12	60–100	100–120

Disability
GCS score cannot be applied to children under 5 years – use AVPU or a Paediatric GCS score.

Exposure
Large body surface area = prone to hypothermia.

Non-accidental injury

- Consider the possibility of NAI in children presenting with the following:
- Injury not consistent with history given.
- Not possible in age of child (e.g. cannot walk).
- Changing or vague history.
- Delay in seeking medical attention.
- Lack of parental concern.
- Frequent Emergency department attendances.
- Multiple fractures of different ages.
- Rib fractures with history of low mechanism of injury.
- Long bone fractures in children <3 years.

Obtain a senior opinion if you have any suspicions and involve the Paediatric team.

Management of paediatric trauma

Pre-arrival
- Call the Paediatric team.
- Calculate drug doses and gather equipment based on estimated age.
- Warm up the Resuscitation room.

Airway with cervical spine control
- Talk to the patient and assess their response. Listen for any noisy breathing to suggest an obstructed airway. Look inside the mouth and use suction to remove any foreign bodies or debris.
- Provide manual in-line stabilization using a hand on either side of the patients head to hold the neck in a neutral position, or use a cervical collar, blocks, and tape to immobilize the cervical spine. Do not restrain any combative children.
- Use a jaw thrust or basic adjuncts (NPA, OPA) to open the airway. Call for senior Emergency department or Anaesthetic support if the airway is compromised.

Breathing
- 15 L O_2 via a mask with a non-rebreath reservoir bag.
- Count the respiratory rate.
- Examine the chest and treat for any injury.
- Ventilate patients using a bag-valve-mask with a pressure limiter if self-ventilation is inadequate.

Circulation with haemorrhage control
- Assess radial pulse, pulse rate, a central capillary refill, and BP using an appropriately-sized cuff.
- Identify and control any external bleeding.
- Examine the abdomen, pelvis, and femurs for any injury.
- If intravenous access is unsuccessful, use intra-osseous access.
- Use paediatric blood bottles to prevent iatrogenic hypovolaemia!
- Use fluid resuscitation with 20 mL/kg boluses of crystalloid if there is any clinical suspicion of shock, e.g. tachycardia or hypotension. Use blood early or after 40 mL/kg has been administered.

Disability
- Assess GCS (using the Paediatric score for <5 years) and pupils.
- **Don't Ever Forget Glucose (DEFG):** check BM and treat if < 3 mmol with 10 % glucose 5 mL/kg. Caution, this concentration may be irritant especially if extravasation occurs.
- Safely log roll the patient off the spinal board if appropriate. Check the back for any wounds, and palpate down the thoracic and lumbar spine for any tenderness in a conscious patient. Check anal tone and sensation if there is any suspicion of spinal injury.

Exposure
- Undress the patient to allow full examination and identification of any other injuries.
- Keep warm.
- Cover wounds, apply splints.
- Give analgesia.

Options for analgesia

- Paracetamol oral = 20 mg/kg up to 6 hourly.
- Ibuprofen oral = 5 mg/kg. (Not licensed for use in children under 3 months or body-weight under 5 kg).
- Morphine oral solution (oramorph) = 0.2–0.4 mg/kg
- Intranasal diamorphine = 0.1 mg/kg (unlicensed use).
- Morphine IV = 0.1 mg/kg

Please check all drugs with which you are unfamiliar in the BNF or local protocol. Refer to the BNF for further doses and information.

General points

Allow parents or carers to be in the Resuscitation room to comfort the child and identify to you whether the child is behaving normally for them. Explain to the parent what is happening at each stage. Allocate a member of nursing staff to look after the parent.

☠ Trauma in the elderly

Advanced age (>65 years) is associated with a poor outcome for trauma patients. The elderly are up to five times more likely to die after trauma (from multi-organ failure and sepsis) than younger patients.

Mechanism of injury

- Consider if the trauma was actually caused by a medical problem, e.g. a stroke or heart attack?
- Falls are associated with a higher severity of injury.
- RTC car occupants or pedestrians.
- Burns.
- Consider possibility of elder abuse.

Differences in anatomy and physiology in the elderly

The elderly have pre-existing medical conditions, reduced functional capacity of organ systems and polypharmacy.

Airway

- Reduced mouth opening, reduced neck mobility.
- More difficult to BVM as edentulous.
- Very fragile nasal muscosa requiring care when using NPA.

Breathing

- Less reserve due to ageing and chronic lung disease.
- Use caution in giving 15 L O_2 to patients with chronic obstructive pulmonary disease (COPD), which may lead to CO_2 retention. Check the pO_2 and pCO_2 levels on an ABG and alter the inspired oxygen level accordingly.
- Poor expectoration requiring admission for more minor chest injuries.

Circulation

- Less cardiovascular reserves and underlying coronary artery disease.
- Unable to mount the same tachycardia or vasoconstriction in hypovolaemia.
- Blood pressure increases with age so SBP 120 mmHg may be low compared with their normal of 180 mmHg.
- Medications affect response, e.g. beta blockers.
- Early invasive monitoring may be required.

Disability

Atrophic brain with increase risk of subdural bleeds, may be on warfarin/anticoagulants.

Exposure

Prone to hypothermia.

Other
- Osteoporosis and less muscle mass with increased likelihood of fractures.
- Fragile skin and high risk for pressure sores.
- Titrate IV morphine more slowly, avoid regular NSAIDs in the elderly, and consider renal function pre-contrast scan or before giving nephrotoxic antibiotics.
- Tetanus vaccination will often not be up to date.

Making decisions

Advanced patient age alone should not be used as the sole criteria for denying or limiting the level of care provided.

A social history from the patient, relatives, or carers is essential at the earliest opportunity to establish quality of life, normal function, and normal conscious level.

In very elderly patients it is important to assess the patient's capacity and discuss the plan with the patient where possible. In cases where the patient does not have capacity, check whether they have a living will/advanced directive or Lasting Power of Attorney who has been nominated to make decisions for them. Always act in the patients best interests.

:⚙: Burns

Burns are potentially life-threatening injuries, and require a rapid assessment, resuscitation, and referral to a specialist burns unit where appropriate.

History
- Any explosion? Risk of blast injury.
- Any confined space? Risk of CO poisoning and smoke inhalation.
- Duration of exposure?
- Any loss of consciousness?
- Any jump or fall to escape from fire? Risk of traumatic injury.
- PMH? Are they a smoker? Reflects comorbidities and carboxyhaemoglobin (COHb) levels

Depth of burn
Remember that a burn is a dynamic wound and the depth will change according to the effectiveness of resuscitation. There will often be more than one depth of burn within the same area.
- **Superficial:** epidermis only. Erythema, looks like sunburn.
- **Partial thickness – superficial:** epidermis into upper layers of dermis. Blisters, blanches, but regains colour slowly, painful.
- **Partial thickness – deep:** epidermis into deeper layers of dermis. Blisters, mottled red capillary staining, does not blanch, less painful.
- **Full thickness:** dry leathery wound, does not blanch, no sensation, no bleeding on pin prick.

Estimating burn area
There are several commonly used methods of estimating burn area. These include:
- **Palmar surface:** palm of patients hand including fingers represents 1% of their body surface area. Useful for small burns or large burns, in which case measure the unburnt skin.
- **Wallace rule of nines:** body divided into areas of 9% and added together (rule of 10's for children).
- **Lund and Browder chart:** shade area on a chart and add the percentages together. Useful for children as it allows for variation in body ratios with age (see Fig. 8.2).

Inhalational injury
Inhalational injury should be suspected if there is:
- Singed facial hair.
- Soot in nostrils or on palate.
- Carbonaceous sputum.
- Burns to face or neck.
- Hoarse voice or stridor.
- Unconscious or confused.

The risks are of impending oedema with upper airway obstruction, chemical lung injury with respiratory failure, and poisoning with carbon monoxide or cyanide.

Fluid resuscitation

Burns greater than 10% total body surface area (TBSA) in children or >15% TBSA in adults require intravenous fluid resuscitation with crystalloid.

Parkland formula

$$4 \times TBSA \% \times weight\ in\ kg = amount\ of\ fluid\ in\ 24\ h$$

Give the first half in the first 8 h and the other half in the next 16 h.

The calculated volume starts from time of injury. Therefore, delete the amount of administered pre-hospital fluid from the total and ensure the administration rate will make up for any deficits from the time of injury.

Monitor adequacy of resuscitation by urine output: a minimum of 0.5 mg/kg/h in adults and 1 mg/kg/h in children. May require higher urine outputs if there is any biochemical evidence of rhabdomyolysis from extensive or deep burns.

Non-accidental injury in children

Unintentional burns and scalds are common in childhood, and these should all be referred to the paediatric liaison nurse for the hospital or the child's health visitor/school nurse, to allow education on accident prevention. A minority of burns may be caused by NAI and some of the high risk signs include:
- Late presentation.
- History does not fit injury pattern.
- Child's age does not fit with injury pattern.
- Stocking and glove distribution scalds suggestive of immersion in water.
- Circular deep burns consistent with the size of a cigarette end.
- Other unexplained injuries.

Seek senior Paediatric advice if you have any suspicions.

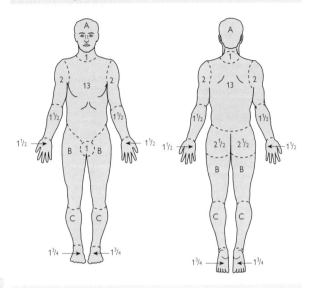

Relative percentage of area affected by growth (age in years)

	0	1	5	10	15	Adult
A: half of head	9½	8½	6½	5½	4½	3½
B: half of thigh	2¾	3¼	4	4½	4½	4¾
C: half of leg	2½	2½	2¾	3	3¼	3½

Fig. 8.2 Assessing extent of burns – Lund and Browder charts. Reproduced from Wyatt *et al.* (2006), with permission from Oxford University Press.

Burns management

Airway
Assess for airway burns and call senior anaesthetist early. Re-evaluate regularly for non-intubated patients.

C- spine
Immobilize the spine if there is any history of significant trauma escaping from fire or blast injury

Breathing
- Give 15 L oxygen immediately.
- Assess chest for injury.
- Treat any wheeze with salbutamol 5 mg nebulized in oxygen.
- Check ABG for CO levels (normal < 10% in smokers, lower in non-smokers), and adequacy of oxygenation and ventilation
- Request a CXR.
- Consider other effects from smoke inhalation, e.g. cyanide.
- Full thickness burns, which are circumferential to chest may restrict chest wall movements and require escharotomy by a trained surgeon.

Circulation
- Identify any associated injuries to abdomen, pelvis, femurs etc which can cause hypovolaemic shock (burns rarely cause shock in the first couple of hours).
- IV access: try to avoid burnt skin.
- Send bloods for FBC, U&E, creatinine kinase (CK), clotting, G&S
- Commence intravenous fluids according to resuscitation formula.
- Insert urinary catheter and monitor hourly urine output.
- ECG in case of carbon monoxide poisoning to identify arrhythmia or ischaemia.

Disability
Consider head injury or inhalational injury as causes of reduced GCS.

Exposure
- Check the burn has been cooled with cold water or dressing, remove any wet dressings, assess the size and depth of the burn, and cover with cling film.
- Check the neurovascular status of any limbs with burns.
- Remove any constricting jewellery or clothing.
- Keep the patient warm with blankets/bear hugger and avoid hypothermia.

Burn wound management
- Analgesia, e.g. IV morphine titrated to pain.
- Loosely cover burn with cling film, avoiding circumferential wrapping.
- Check tetanus status and give booster as necessary.
- Prophylactic antibiotics are not indicated in the early management.
- Speak to the Regional Burns team as early as possible to discuss specific treatment.

Chemical burns

The severity of a chemical burn is related to the product, the concentration, and the duration of contact. Patients who have suffered industrial burns should bring an information sheet with them from the company regarding the type of chemical.

The treatment involves continuous irrigation with large amounts of water and removal of any contaminated clothes. Remember to avoid contaminating yourself and wear appropriate protective equipment. Obtain advice from the National Poisons Units or TOXBASE regarding any particular antidotes for named domestic or industrial products.

❶ Referral to a specialist burns unit
This is indicated if there is any evidence of:
- Airway burns/inhalational injury.
- Full thickness burns >1%.
- Burns >10% TBSA in children and >15% TBSA in adults.
- Burns in special areas, e.g. face, hands, feet, joints, genitals.
- Circumferential burns.
- Complex electrical burns or chemical burns.

Reference

Wyatt, J., et al. (2006) *Oxford Handbook of Emergency Medicine*, 3rd edn. Oxford: Oxford University Press.

☠ Electrical injury

Electrical injury causes pathology by depolarizing muscles and nerves, producing arrhythmias, or producing internal and external burns (with tissue damage often more extensive than the visible surface burns). Common mechanisms of injury include children or DIY at home; industrial injury, train circuits, or lightning strikes on the golf course.

Types of electrical injury
- Low voltage AC, e.g. domestic 230 V.
- High voltage AC, e.g. industrial or power line >1000 V.
- High voltage DC, e.g. lightning strike.

Factors determining the severity of electrical injury
- Voltage.
- Type of current, e.g. AC worse than DC.
- Duration of contact.
- Path of current, e.g. across chest or head worse.
- Resistance of tissues, e.g. bone > muscle > blood vessels > nerves.
- Associated injury, e.g. falls.

Potential sequelae from electrical injury
- **Cardiac arrhythmias or cardiac arrest** [ventricular fibrillation (VF) with AC, asystole with DC].
- **Muscle injury:**
  - leading to myonecrosis, swelling, and compartment syndrome of limbs;
  - leading to rhabdomyolysis and renal failure.
- **Burns:**
  - *flash burns* – usually superficial as shock passes over surface of body;
  - *arc* – deep partial thickness/full thickness, worse if clothing ignites;
  - *direct contact entry and exit burns* – often full thickness.
- **Injuries** from falls or involuntary contraction of muscles causing fracture-dislocations.
- **Neurological complications**, including seizures, transient paralysis, loss of consciousness, and peripheral neuropathy.
- **Eye complications** (particularly post-lightening strike to head), e.g. glaucoma or cataract.

Management

- Commence CPR if patient is in cardiac arrest.
- Airway including a check for burns of the mouth or oropharynx, which may cause oedema and airway obstruction.
- Examine BCD for any life threatening injury.
- Commence fluids if severe electrical injury or any myoglobinuria and maintain a urine output of 1–2 mL/kg/h. (The standard burns formula will under predict fluid requirements.)
- Expose fully to inspect for any burns to the skin.
- Check distal pulses and sensation in limbs.

Investigations

- 12-lead ECG.
- Send bloods including FBC, U&E, and a CK.
- Check urine for blood on dipstick, which may indicate myoglobinuria. If sample is positive send to the laboratory for verification (absence of red cells).
- ABG.

Specific treatment

- Admit all symptomatic patients.
- Senior orthopaedic review for any swollen limb injuries with a risk of compartment syndrome.
- Refer any significant burns to the local burns centre for specialist opinion/transfer.

Discharge post-electrical injury

The following criteria must all be present to allow safe discharge:
- Low voltage domestic electrical injury.
- No loss of consciousness.
- Normal ECG, and no chest pain or palpitations.
- No blood on urine dipstick.
- No burns or other injuries requiring admission.

:☻: **Blast injury**

Mechanism of injury
- Gas explosion.
- Industrial explosion.
- Terrorist bomb.

Classification of injuries
Primary blast injury
Injuries due to the interaction of the shock wave with the body causing:
- Lung injury, e.g. pneumothorax, pulmonary contusion.
- Tympanic membrane perforation (not an indicator of severity of blast injury).
- Bowel contusions and perforations.
- Cerebral and coronary air embolism.
- Traumatic amputations.

The severity of the primary blast injury is worse in a confined space or underwater, and with closer proximity to the explosion.

Secondary blast injury
Fragmentation injury from the bomb material or flying debris causing penetrating injury or lacerations.

Tertiary blast injury
Victim is thrown by blast wind and suffers traumatic injuries on landing.

Other
- Burns and smoke inhalation.
- Crush injury.
- Psychological.
- Infection from contamination by human tissue/blood, e.g. suicide bombers.

Management
- ABCD assessment. Examine the lungs and abdomen carefully for all patients involved in a significant explosion. Remember the patient is at high risk of pneumothorax/tension pneumothorax if intubation and ventilation is required.
- CXR if any respiratory symptoms or signs.
- FAST scan if there is any abdominal pain or haemodynamic instability. A negative scan may need to be followed by a CT abdomen to detect acute intestinal perforation.
- Treat penetrating wounds, blunt injuries, or burns as standard. Secondary fragmentation injury is treated comparable with a low velocity GSW. Consider the infection risk of penetrating injuries by other victims blood or tissue, e.g. tetanus, hepatitis B vaccination, HIV PEP, etc.
- Examine the ears during the secondary survey to identify perforated tympanic membranes or haemotympanum.

Who to send home

In a major incident setting it will not be possible to admit every patient for observation.

Admit all patients who were within close proximity to the blast, or in the same room or enclosed space, e.g. bus or train carriage.

For all other patients send home those who are completely asymptomatic, with no obvious injuries and normal vital signs after 4 h of observation. They should be instructed to return immediately to the emergency department if they have any shortness of breath, chest pain, abdominal pain, vomiting, or other symptoms. Remember that pulmonary contusion and bowel haematomas/perforation can take up to 48 h to develop.

Isolated perforated tympanic membrane injuries can be discharged with the advice of avoiding water/drops in the ear and with out-patient ENT follow-up.

All pregnant women exposed to an explosion regardless of the absence of injuries should be examined by the Obstetric team and admitted for observation.

Pitfalls

- Often no external signs of injury in blast lung or abdomen.
- Not checking the eyes of unconscious patients for foreign bodies from fragmentation.
- Not admitting symptomatic patients for observation who are at risk of blast lung or abdominal injury.

Part 2

Orthopaedics

General principles

⑦ General principles

Dealing with a trauma patient whilst on-call requires a high level of organization. Trauma patients range from the medically unwell, e.g. neck of femur fracture patients and polytrauma patients, to the walking wounded who want to go home. Patients are often discharged and brought back to fracture clinics – the skill is knowing who is safe to send home and when to bring them back.

Who is safe for home?
- Those who can get home without driving.
- Those who have someone at home to look after them.
- Those who can come back to Fracture Clinic.

Who is not safe for home?
- Those living alone (complications may develop at home).
- Unreliable patients (e.g. those who will return to work and not rest).
- Those at high risk of developing compartment syndrome, e.g. displaced, closed tibial fractures.
- Those requiring elevation and immobilization, e.g. swollen ankle fractures requiring open reduction, internal fixation (ORIF).
- Those with significant co-morbidity (e.g. COPD and chest wall injury).
- Those at risk – deliberate self-harm, those prone to abuse (the family may be the abuser).

For immediate surgery
- For example, open fracture, polytrauma, traumatic amputations.
- Assess for acute trauma bed. Consider sick/unstable patients for HDU/ITU.

For surgery, list available tomorrow
- Admitting the patient is the easiest and most reliable method.
- Reliable, young patients (e.g. requiring wrist surgery tomorrow) can come back for 08.00 the next morning, starved if a bed can be guaranteed (liaise with bed manager).
- Book on the *trauma list* before they go home.
- Take the patient's phone number yourself in case of change.
- If likely for surgery (but not definite) and able to go home [e.g. children for manipulation under anaesthesia (MUA) with borderline distal radius fracture], send home, give instructions to starve that night, discuss at the morning trauma meeting and inform patient (they can then come in, starved if necessary).

For surgery, no list today/tomorrow
- Send home if safe (e.g. young patient needing 5th metacarpal surgical reduction).
- Ensure the patient has adequate and enough analgesia.
- Get contact details (mobile and landline) and add to the *rolling trauma list* (the list for those waiting for surgery).
- Arrange for patient to come back in starved when a list and surgeon is available.

Not for surgery, not safe for home
- For example, an elderly lady with a proximal humerus fracture, who lives alone. Admit for social reasons.
- A rehabilitation bed is preferable over an acute trauma bed, if available. Access to this may be directly through Emergency department (ED) or physicians.
- If in doubt, admit under your care for safety.

Not for surgery, safe for home
- Discharge with advice, analgesia, and follow-up.
- Make sure follow-up is arranged (Fracture Clinic).
- Arrange a visit to the next suitable Fracture Clinic if in doubt.

Preparing trauma patients for surgery
- Decide what operation is needed. The consultant has the final say.
- **Consent:** only if you know how the procedure is performed and the potential complications.
- **Mark:** mark the side of surgery with an arrow using a *permanent* marker. Mark away from the site of incision. For fingers, mark the forearm and mark the relevant fingernail.
- **NBM:** see below. Inform the patient and nurses.
- **Bloods:** FBC, U&E for the elderly or for moderate/large procedures. G&S/cross-match for procedure specific.
- Consider ECG and CXR as appropriate.
- **Fluids:** trauma patients, even those with simple fractures, are often dehydrated. Good hydration helps prevent complications, such as deep vein thrombosis (DVT)/acute renal failure. Consider intravenous infusion (IVI), especially whilst NBM.
- **Medical reviews:** you should be able to start initial management of acute medical conditions (e.g. antibiotics, nebulizers, and chest physiotherapy for chest infections), although early review by a medical registrar is good practice. This is often easier whilst the patient is in the ED.
- Book on the trauma list. Inform the anaesthetist early if there is a problem (e.g. significant medical comorbidities).
- **Starve** solid food 6 h prior to surgery, clear fluids 2 h prior (check local policy). No chewing gum (gastric stimulant).

Fracture Clinics

- These are usually run daily.
- Access is often through direct booking from ED.
- Ask for the notes to go to Fracture Clinic.
- If in doubt, bring back to 'next available Fracture Clinic'.
- If in doubt over a fracture and there is no senior available (e.g. 'Is the scaphoid fractured?' 'Is there a small crack of the distal radius?') treat as a fracture and bring back to the next Fracture Clinic. Explain fully to the patient that the treatment may be reversed.
- For injures likely to need an expert, try and get the patient into an appropriate specialist clinic (discuss with that consultant first if possible).

⑦ Assessing the patient with a fracture

Assessing a patient with an isolated fracture is different from assessing a polytraumatized patient as part of a trauma alert, as you will often be alone. Once a referral from the ED has been accepted, you will need to assess and clerk the patient. General principles of history and examination still count, but this section highlights what the orthopaedic on-call doctor needs to consider.

First assessments

Although the ED should have completed a primary and secondary survey, this may have been overlooked with seemingly 'simple' fractures, or the patient's condition may have changed since referral. Thus, approach each patient systematically:

- **ABC:** repeat primary survey and actively seek out occult injuries, which may have been missed.
- **Secondary survey:** despite the obvious injury, check for other areas of pain or injury. Minor fingers injuries, for example, may be missed at this stage, which will cause morbidity unless corrected.
- **Tertiary survey:** the tertiary survey is performed by orthopaedic teams when the patient is on the ward or high dependency units. The patient is fully re-examined again, and further occult trauma and musculoskeletal injuries are sought.

History

Mechanism of injury. Go into detail – 'a fall' is not enough.

- Ask about specific mechanisms, e.g. direction and surface of impact.
- For vehicular accidents, ask about speed, type of car damage, other passenger injuries, seatbelt use, and location within car.
- For falls in the elderly, establish whether it was a mechanical trip, or if there was associated chest pain, breathing difficulties, or loss of consciousness. For the elderly who cannot recall any events, assess for head injuries. Ensure a current ECG is performed, and consider medical review if you cannot identify a cause for the fall.

Examining the fractured/dislocated limb
- **Assess the distal neurovascular status:** loss of pulses is an emergency and may require urgent intervention (e.g. reduction of an ankle dislocation):
  - *pulses* – check all distal pulses are present, e.g. in a child with a supracondylar humeral fracture, check the radial and ulnar pulses are both present;
  - *check the distal neurology* – ensure sensation is intact by checking specific dermatomes.
- **Assess the fracture site:** look for swelling and skin breaks (e.g. open fractures). Check underneath limbs for further injuries. Displaced fractures that have not pierced the skin may still cause 'tenting' of the skin, which will puts tissue viability at high risk; these require urgent reduction (traction in ED is usually enough for the acute phase).
- **Check for swelling:** this may be leading to a compartment syndrome. Very swollen ankles may not be amenable to immediate surgery and should be immobilized, elevated, and treated with ice packs.
- **Clear patients off spinal boards as soon as possible:** they are uncomfortable, stressful, and rapidly lead to pressure sores.
- **Complete cardiovascular, chest, and abdominal examinations** are still mandatory in all patients.
- **Do not forget basics:** document blood pressure, pulse, temperature, bedside glucose, and GCS as a minimum.

Assessing the unconscious patient
- You may be asked to assess an intubated patient, in the Resuscitation room or ITU.
- Quality of primary and secondary survey are even more important, since the patient can no longer report pain:
  - *Examine all bones and joints* – abnormal movements or crepitus may need to be investigated further. X-rays can often wait until the patient is more stable.
  - For unconscious patients with long bone trauma, feel the compartments and check distal pulses, as they cannot report the pain of compartment syndromes. Tense compartments need compartment pressures to be checked.
  - Forearm fractures can be elevated in Bradford slings in ITU to immobilize and prevent further damage. Well fitted backslabs (not too tight or loose) can be applied.
  - Open fractures in this group still require good initial cleaning, photographing and dressing. However, definite debridement may need to be delayed until the patient is more stable.

Plain film radiographs

Although ED physicians will often have undertaken initial X-rays, further X-rays may be required for surgical assessment. It is easier to send patients for further X-rays prior to sending to the ward, rather than bringing them back down.

> The ideal set of radiographs for any fracture or dislocation includes two views, with two joints (that above and below) at two times (pre- and post-reduction).

- If ED have applied an ankle backslab for an unstable ankle fracture, a post-reduction film is needed (the position may have altered).
- For peri-prosthetic fractures, X-rays are needed all the way to the tip of the prosthesis.
- For metastatic fractures, the whole bone needs to be seen at this stage, e.g. full length femur X-rays for suspected pathological fractures of the neck of femur.

Investigations

- **Blood tests:** consider FBC, U&E, clotting (especially if on anticoagulants, liver disease, etc.) and blood grouping as pre-operative blood tests.
- **X-rays:** as above. A chest X-ray is useful for those with chest symptoms and for all fractured neck of femur patients.
- **ECG:** for the pre-operative patient or those with falls and amnesia. It is easier to do these in ED, rather wait till the ward (which may be some hours away).
- **Investigate other systems as appropriate:** place requests for echocardiograms, lung function testing, bone scans, and CT scans as soon as possible (in conjunction with senior and anaesthetic advice).

Initial management

- Adequate resuscitation and analgesia.
- Immobilization helps to prevent pain and limit further soft tissue damage. Backslabs are easy to apply in the ED and are effective. Ensure they are not loose, but not too tight either. Specific splints for bigger injuries may be needed (e.g. Thomas splints for femoral shaft fractures).
- Elevate limbs wherever possible. Hand/wrist/forearm injuries can be elevated in Bradford slings, and ankle/knee injuries on Braun frames or pillows.
- Find out which ward patients are going to and keep a clear list.

The drug chart

When writing up a drug chart for a trauma patient, remember the following:

- **Analgesia:** provide basic regular analgesia (e.g. co-codamol 30/500, two tablets qds; ibuprofen 400 mg tds or diclofenac 50 mg tds [consider gastro-protection with PPI]) and stronger prn analgesia (e.g. Oramorph 5–10 mg, qds).
- Prescribe a prn antiemetic (e.g. cyclizine, 50 mg IM/IV/po).
- For the elderly being started on opiates, prescribe laxatives to prevent constipation (rather than waiting until it happens).
- **DVT prophylaxis:** most lower limb or immobile trauma patients should receive low weight molecular heparin (e.g. enoxaparin, 40 mg sc od) and possibly TEDS. Be guided by local policies.
- **Regular medications:** consider what needs to be given and omitted, e.g. warfarin may need to be temporarily stopped pre-operatively.

Talking to the patient/family

- Give information as required, without being too specific unless you are sure (this may be best left to senior team members). Don't tell the patient they need an operation if they might not, as this makes future communication difficult.
- If you are able to take consent, do it now and ask the patient to sign the consent form. If you are not sure what the operation entails or how to take consent, leave it to someone senior (but communicate that it needs to be done).
- Communicate with family, especially of the elderly and children.

Do not communicate facts that you are unsure about. Seek senior advice first.

⑦ **Interpreting and describing X-rays**

Knowing how to interpret and then describe bony X-rays is important, not only so you know what you're dealing with (and that you're not missing anything), but also as you may have to describe this over the phone to an orthopaedic consultant. Even if a bone is not fractured, there may be problems with joints (e.g. arthritis or dislocations), soft tissue, or foreign bodies.

Ensure the correct X-rays

- Ensure the correct X-rays are present – correct patient, correct side, adequate views (i.e. two views are needed or assessment of most fractures/dislocations, joint above and below for every long bone fracture).
- Ensure you have seen the patient before discussing the X-rays. You cannot tell if a fracture is open or if there is vascular compromise from the X-ray, nor whether the patient will be fit for an operation.

Interpreting

- Interpreting the X-rays without having seen the patient is difficult and potentially dangerous. Make your own clinical assessment, to include whether the fracture is open or closed, vascular injuries, compartment syndromes, swelling of the soft tissues, and general medical conditions.
- The ABCs system is easy to remember and use:
  - A – *Adequacy and Alignment* – adequacy relates to enough of the involved bone or joint, e.g. joint above and below in every long bone fracture. From C1 to C7/T1 junction for a lateral cervical spine. From the top of the iliac crest to the proximal femur for a pelvis. Alignment relates to the contours of adjacent bones, identifying steps caused by fractures and dislocations.
  - B – *Bone margins and density* – check outline of each bone, looking for breaks and bends in the cortex indicating fractures. Once the main abnormality has been seen, look systematically around all other bones to check for more subtle injuries (especially for the foot and hand). Check the bone looking for abnormalities (that may indicate pathological fractures caused by osteoporosis or malignancy).
  - C – *Cartilage and joints* – changes in cartilage spaces (such as those between vertebrae and joints) suggest fracture or dislocations.
  - S – *Soft tissues* – swelling, tissue loss, foreign bodies.

Describing

- **Open or closed:** state this early as the management is different and this conveys the urgency.
- **Bone involved:** name the main bone involved and then any others. Fit in a description of the fracture position within the bone, e.g. proximal, middle, or distal third.
- **Pattern:** pick the most appropriate of the different types: transverse, oblique, spiral, comminuted (more than two fragments), wedge (e.g. osteoporotic wedge fracture of a vertebrae), avulsion, pathological, or greenstick (children) (see Fig. 9.1).

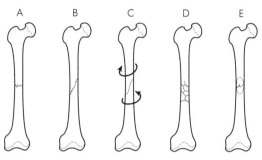

Fig. 9.1 Patterns of fractures. A. Transverse; B. Oblique; C. Spiral; D. Comminuted; E. Pathological.

- **Deformity:** is defined in several ways (Fig. 9.2):
  - *displacement* – the percentage loss of end-to-end contact of the proximal and distal ends (e.g. there is 50% dorsal displacement of the distal end of the radius);
  - *shortening* – if occurring, to what extent [e.g. the distal radius has shortened (*or impacted*) by approximately 2 cm].
  - *angulation* – of the distal to proximal ends (e.g. the degree of dorsal angulation of the distal radius with a Colles fracture);
  - *rotation* – of the distal portion relative to the proximal portion; this should be correlated with clinical findings (e.g. with metacarpal fractures).
- **Intra-articular involvement:** mention early if the fracture extends into a joint (look at the intra-articular surface for gaps, breaks, and steps). If it has, mention whether the intra-articular component is comminuted (e.g. the articular surface is multi-fragmented) and the size of step. Displaced intra-articular fractures often need ORIF to prevent a loss of function.
- **Dislocations:** if this is a fracture-dislocation, mention early. Describe both the fracture and the dislocation (e.g. there is an anterior dislocation of the shoulder with a displaced fracture of the greater tuberosity).

- **Associations:** mention any gross soft tissue swelling, other injuries, damage to tendons, general medical condition. Ensure you confirm whether the distal neurovascular status is intact or not; vascular/ neurological compromise requires urgent senior review, and you should mention any suspicion of compartment syndrome (established or impending) early on.
- Mention relevant information that alters management, e.g. metal allergies, significant medical co-morbidities.

Discussing treatment

- Mention what has already been done (such as analgesia, application of backslabs) and what else you will do.
- If you have a specific question, ask it now.

Then await further instructions on management.

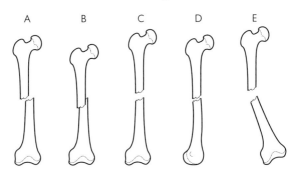

A   B   C   D   E

Fig. 9.2 Deformities of fractures. A. Displacement; B. Shortening; C. Distraction; D. Rotation; E. Angulation. Adapted from a figure published by Bhangu & Keighley (2007). © Elsevier 2007.

Pitfalls

- Not having reviewed the patient clinically before discussing X-rays with seniors.
- If you have not seen the patient, but are required to discuss them with seniors, make it clear this is the case at the outset (although always do try to see the patient first!).
- Focusing on the obvious fracture and missing smaller, but equally important second or third injuries.
- Failing to consider soft tissue injuries, as well as the broken bone.

Example

This is a closed fracture of the distal radius in a 70-year-old woman. There is no neurovascular compromise. It is comminuted and intra-articular. There is 50% dorsal displacement, with approximately 2 cm of shortening. There is an intra-articular step of approximately 3 mm. There is no significant past medical history or co-morbidities. I plan to place the forearm in a backslab and admit this patient for a volar locking plate.

Reference

Bhangu, A., & Keighley, M. (2007) *The Flesh and Bones of Surgery*. Oxford: Elsevier.

☼ Open fractures

Open fractures are orthopaedic emergencies, where the aim of treatment is to prevent a contaminated wound from becoming an infected wound. An open fracture may be an isolated injury or part of a polytraumatized patient. The use of the term *compound* has caused confusion in the past; *open* or *closed* provides unambiguous, clear terminology.

Types of open fracture

- Open fractures may range from partial amputations to 'in-out' puncture wounds.
- Open femoral fractures typically occur after high speed RTCs and are associated with large volume blood loss and other injuries.
- **Traumatic amputations:** in the presence of massive external bleeding, blood loss should be controlled by the immediate use of a tourniquet; this is the C-ABC paradigm. For injuries without massive external bleeding, by definition, bleeding is not immediately life-threatening (and so should be addressed under the C of ABC). For most wounds, direct pressure, appropriate dressing, and elevation will arrest haemorrhage.
- **'In/out' wounds** typically occur around the lower leg and ankle, and the protruding bone, and sometimes a small relieving incision is necessary to relocate protruding bone. In this case senior advice should be immediately obtained.
- **Protruding bone:** again common with long bones, the patient should be rapidly treated and traction may be needed to replace the protruding bone back into the body.
- **Open joint injuries:** although there may be no fracture, these are treated in the same way.
- **Fractures with soft tissue injury:** an underlying fracture that has not displaced, but which communicates with the skin due to soft tissue loss is treated as an open fracture. A fracture with an overlying superficial graze can be treated as a closed fracture. If in doubt, treat as open and get a senior opinion.

Examination and investigation

- ABC principles apply as for assessing any trauma patient.
- Check carefully for occult injuries (local and distant), distal pulses, and compartment syndrome.
- Check X-rays for foreign bodies (show glass and metal, but not grit/dirt).

Management

- Try and get to the ED before the wound has been dressed or covered, as once covered it should not be uncovered. You will need to be quick; don't ask them to delay for you.
- There are four key aims in the ED:
  - *Initial debridement* – before more thorough surgical debridement. Wash thoroughly and copiously with sodium chloride 0.9%, and remove large pieces of debris, without causing excessive pain or damaging tissue. Local anaesthetic may be needed (e.g. ring blocks for fingers).
  - *Photograph* – prior to dressing, which can be shown to seniors, rather than constantly undressing the wound (and, hence, introducing more infection).
  - *Dress* – dress and cover the wound. For the first layer use either povidone-iodine-soaked gauze or Inadine dressings. Pad with more gauze, and wrap with a firm crepe bandage.
  - *Antibiotics* – the patient should be started on intravenous antibiotics according to local protocols, and tetanus status checked and updated. First doses should be given before the patient leaves ED. Surgical debridement is better than immunization at preventing tetanus infection.
- For large/unstable fractures, a temporary backslab can be applied. Patients should be NBM, admitted to a ward, and prepared for theatre.
- X-rays should be taken.
- Orthopaedic teams need to be called early in the ED. Surgical options depend on the fracture and quality of tissues. Dirty, contaminated wounds can be left open, with a second look and debridement at 48 h. Large skin losses may need plastic surgery input. Small, clean wounds whose skin edges come together tension free can be closed primarily.
- Aim to get the patient to an operating theatre within 6 h.

Classification

The Gustilo (and Anderson) Classification is useful for communicating with colleagues over the phone:

- **Grade I:** wound <1 cm, moderately clean, simple fracture pattern.
- **Grade II:** wound >1 cm without extensive soft tissue damage or loss, and there is moderate contamination and comminution.
- **Grade III:** extensive damage to soft tissues, highly contaminated, fracture often comminuted, associated vascular injuries, traumatic amputations, high velocity injuries:
  - *type A* – the wound can be closed using simple means;
  - *type B* – a flap is required;
  - *type C* – presence of a vascular injury requiring repair.

Pitfalls

- Missing life-threatening injuries by not performing a full primary and secondary survey.
- Failure to get the patient to theatre with due haste.
- Repeatedly uncovering the wound.

☠: **Compartment syndrome**

Compartment syndrome of a limb is a time-dependant orthopaedic emergency. It occurs when pressure within a muscular fascial compartment exceeds tissue perfusion pressure, leading to muscle and nerve ischaemia. Although typically associated with fractures of the tibia, it may occur elsewhere and also in the absence of fractures, when factors such as tissue damage and drugs cause compartment swelling.

Pathology

- Swelling within a closed fascial compartment impedes venous outflow. As intra-compartmental pressure rises further, venous outflow blockade eventually impedes arterial inflow. Ischaemia leads to muscle necrosis. Nerves also undergo ischaemic changes.
- Compartment syndrome may be immediate or delayed, sometimes over 24 h from time of injury.

Predisposing factors

- **Fractures:** both open and closed. Open fractures may breach the fascia and thus relieve the pressure.
- **Tight bandages and plaster casts:** these may be well fitted when applied, but continued swelling may occur.
- **Soft tissue damage:** e.g. a collapsed patient who has been lying on their side/limbs whilst on a hard floor for a prolonged period.
- **Crush injuries:** with associated rhabdomyolysis.
- **Incorrect positioning during surgery:** leading to undue pressure on limbs.
- **Administration of chemotherapy:** e.g. through arm lines.

Associated fractures

- **Calf:** tibial fractures (more often in closed fractures, but can also occur with open fractures and should not be overlooked).
- **Foot:** calcaneal/forefoot fractures.
- **Forearm:** radius/ulna fractures.
- **Hand/wrist:** crush injuries.

Signs and symptoms

- **Pain:** is the first and key sign. Pain within a compartment that is out of proportion to signs or that is worsening. The patient cannot get comfortable in any position and is in 'agony'.
- Pain that is worsened by passively flexing the compartment, e.g. with calf compartment syndrome, dorsiflexion of the big toe (pushing the toe up) dramatically worsens the pain as does moving the fingers for the hand/forearm.
- Pain that is unresponsive to opiate analgesia (i.e. morphine).
- The affected compartment may be swollen and discoloured.
- **Silent compartment syndrome:** consider in the unconscious (e.g. intubated). Tense compartments may be palpable; compartment pressures may be needed. May also occur in those with regional/spinal anaesthesia, where progressive neurology is found.

- **Check for pulses and compare the opposite uninjured side for quality:** pulses are often present with a compartment syndrome; pulselessness is a late sign.
- Pallor, paralysis, and parasthesia are late signs.
- Left untreated, irreversible muscle damage may occur at 4–6 h, and pain may decrease.
- Complications include life-threatening rhabdomyolysis (with subsequent acute renal failure) and limb-threatening Volkmann's ischaemic contractures.

Investigations

- A clinical diagnosis is adequate.
- Compartment pressures give an objective measurement:
  - specific hand-held pressure transducers are available;
  - best measured close to fracture (within 5 cm);
  - diastolic blood pressure minus compartment pressure should be >30 mmHg;
  - at 30 mmHg or below, fasciotomy is indicated.
- ABG assesses acidosis from tissue loss/necrosis.
- Serum creatinine kinase is raised from muscular damage. Urgent serum potassium should be checked in cases of rhabdomyolysis and life-threatening hyperkalaemia corrected.
- Urine dipstick may be positive for 'blood' signifying rhabdomyolysis from crush injuries. Urine cytology identifies myoglobinuria.

Management

- **If a plaster cast/backslab is the culprit, open it immediately.** Split the cast, release down to skin (including cotton wool layers, which may continue applying pressure) and split open backslabs, so relieving direct pressure on the muscle group (e.g. the calf).
- Elevate the affected limb at heart level (not above, which decreases arterial flow).
- Administer IV fluids to correct hypoperfusion and oliguria.
- Urgent fasciotomy in an operating theatre is needed for other cases. Inform seniors early. Ensure perioperative hydration and correction of acidosis.
- Rhabdomyolysis with subsequent acute renal failure may develop. Ensure hydration with fluid resuscitation. Forced alkaline diuresis may be used to prevent ferrihaemate pigment renal damage (in critical care settings).

Pitfalls

- Low clinical suspicion ('it's just some pain from the fracture').
- Failing to split backslabs down to skin, including cotton-wool layers.
- Waiting until the compartment syndrome establishes, rather than treating to prevent.

:☠: Fat embolism syndrome

All patients with significant long bone fractures experience some degree of fat embolism. Some progress to fat embolism syndrome and this is related to the number of long bone fractures, failure to correct hypovolaemia and hypoxia, and delays in immobilizing fractures.

Pathology
- Mechanical theories describe fractures of long bones or reaming of intramedullary canals releasing fat globules into the circulation.
- These reach and occlude the small arterioles of the lungs.
- Respiratory failure occurs, and may progress to adult respiratory distress syndrome (ARDS).
- More common in fractures treated conservatively. Thus, early fixation of long bone fractures may be preventative.
- Biochemical theories describe hormonal changes associated with trauma and sepsis as causative.

Predisposing factors
- Multiple bony injuries.
- Delays in resuscitation, including correction of hypoxia and hypovolaemia.
- Poor immobilization of long bone fractures.
- Failure to adhere to damage control orthopaedic principles.

Signs, symptoms, and clinical findings
- Have a high level of suspicion in patients with sudden onset respiratory complications with long bone fractures, especially when occurring within the 72 h of initial trauma.
- **Shortness of breath:** tachypnoea with respiratory distress, ranging from mild to severe.
- Altered level of consciousness, and new, sudden confusion.
- Pyrexia.
- **Fat petechia:** skin (especially axillae) or subconjunctival petechia may be visible.
- Fat globules may be visible in the urine. Fat may also be visible in retinal vessels upon fundoscopy.

Diagnosis
The diagnosis can be made clinically.

To formally diagnose, assess for fat microglobulinaemia (look for fat globules in the urine) and at least one major and four minor signs:
- **Major:** petechial skin rash, hypoxia, confusion without other cause, pulmonary oedema.
- **Minor:** tachycardia, pyrexia, elevated ESR, retinal fat emboli (fundoscopy needed), fat in urine, acute fall in haemoglobin and/or platelets, fat globules in sputum.

Investigations

- ABG reveals hypoxia and assesses the degree of respiratory failure.
- Chest X-ray to help diagnose acute lung injury (ALI) and/or ARDS, and exclude other causes. Serial radiographs to show progressive lung injuries and infiltrates.
- FBC may reveal a fall in haemoglobin and/or platelets, and raised erythrocyte sedimentation rate (ESR). U&E for renal dysfunction.
- Fat globules are found in blood and urine upon microscopy.

Management

- The aims of aggressive management are to ensure perfusion and oxygentation.
- On the ward give high flow oxygen and fluid resuscitation.
- These patients are best managed on ITU; *involve critical care early.*
- IV crystalloids and colloids are used to maintain perfusion.
- Oxygen therapy, including intubation, may be needed to ensure adequate oxygenation.
- Arterial lines allow for serial ABGs; central lines may be needed for closer monitoring.
- Low weight molecular heparin for DVT prophylaxis.
- Proton pump inhibitor (PPI) cover to prevent gastrointestinal stress ulceration.
- Early nutritional support.

Pitfalls

- Low clinical suspicion ('well the sats are only a little low, let's give a little more oxygen and see').
- Once diagnosis made, under-appreciation of severity or potential for deterioration.

:☼: Septic arthritis

Septic arthritis is an orthopaedic emergency that presents in a variety of patients of all ages, in a variety of ways. Recognizing these cases early helps identify those who will benefit from early surgical washout.

Pathology

- Infection within the joint may be from a variety of sources: penetrating trauma, local source (e.g. local abscess, cellulitis, osteomyelitis), distant source (e.g. infection in elderly, blood-borne pathogens), iatrogenic (e.g. post-surgery, post aspiration).
- Diabetics, the immunosuppressed, and extremes of age (very young or very old) are at increased risk.
- The hip is in the most common site in infants (<1 year). In adults the knee is the most common site.
- Overall, *Staphylococcus aureus* accounts for 90% of cases. Special cases include:
  - *Neisseria gonorrhoeae* – the most common cause of septic arthritis in adults under 30 years; this is a sexually transmitted organism;
  - *Pseudomonas aeruginosa* – implicated with intravenous drug abusers;
  - *Salmonella spp.* – a common cause of osteomyelitis in patients with sickle cell anaemia.
  - *Haemophilus influenza* – incidence has decreased with childhood vaccination.
  - *Staphylococcus epidermidis* – the most common organism in infected total joint replacement.

Signs, symptoms, and clinical findings

- In adults, the knee is classically hot, swollen, and tender. Range of movement in all directions is reduced to only a few degrees. Swelling is hot and tense.
- Hip infection results in flexion and internal rotation.
- In neonates, infants, and children, the child prefers not to use the affected limb, e.g. will stand on the 'good' leg. The child may be generally irritable, unwell, tachycardic, or septic. They may not localize to the hip, so a hip and knee examination should be routine in any young child with a sepsis of unknown origin. Compare the abnormal to normal side in the young.
- Patients may be systemically septic.

Investigations

- FBC [for white cell count (WCC)], CRP, ESR, clotting (those on warfarin may have a mimicking haemarthrosis), U&E (pre-operative).
- CXR/ECG as necessary for pre-operative assessment.
- X-rays: AP and lateral to look for fractures and changes of osteomyelitis. Often normal in early disease.
- **Aspiration and culture is the key investigation:** this allows immediate inspection of the type of swelling (e.g. frank blood, pus, serous effusion) and immediate microscopy. Send in a sterile universal specimen pot. No matter the hour, inform the microbiology technician that an urgent sample is on its way as they may not be onsite during the night. During the day they can have an initial result in hours, overnight they can be waiting for the sample in the morning.
- Frank pus on aspiration is an indication for washout. Aspiration on the ward/ED is suitable for knees, shoulders, elbows, wrists, and ankles. Hip aspiration should be undertaken in theatre under image intensifier. Aspiration in young children may need a GA.
- Avoid aspiration through cellulitic skin. A needle through the cellulitis may introduce infection into a normal joint.

Management

- Keep all patients NBM until senior review. Cover with IV fluids. Not all patients will need immediate theatre, although this should be a senior-led decision.
- Aspiration is both diagnostic and therapeutic.
- For frank septic arthritis, formal washout under general anaesthetic (GA) in theatre is needed. Prepare the patient and warn theatre.
- Give IV fluids in the dehydrated with enoxaprin cover.
- Give antibiotics **after** joint aspirate has been obtained. Start with 'best guess', adjust to earliest sensitivities.
- Beware a flushed unwell patient, with tachycardia and pyrexia.

Septic arthritis in those with prosthetic joints

- Infection in a joint with a prosthesis [e.g. following total knee replacement) may present as early infection (weeks) to late infection (years)].
- There may be an absence of pain, since metal joint surfaces convey no nerves. Because of this, movement may be preserved. A discharging sinus over the joint is very suspicious.
- Aspiration for those with prosthetic implants should be done *only* in an operating theatre under sterile conditions (not ED).

Pitfalls

- Giving antibiotics before aspiration (masks culture results).
- Aspirating prosthetic joints in the ED.
- Incomplete examinations of un-operative, septic children.

Differential diagnosis

- **Adults:** gout, reactive arthritis, overlying cellulitis, osteomyelitis.
- **Children:** irritable hip, Perthes disease, osteomyelitis.

⑦ **Aspirating a knee**

The knee is the most common joint that will require aspiration in the emergency department and on the wards. However, since you will be penetrating the joint, introducing an infection is a complication and, therefore, aspiration should be undertaken as a sterile procedure (see Fig. 9.3).

Indications

- **Diagnostic:** in suspected cases of septic arthritis.
- **Therapeutic:** for painful, tense effusions. Good for tender effusions of rheumatoid arthritis and tense haemarthrosis following ligamental injuries (and, occasionally, some fractures around the knee). The risk-benefit must be considered; pain relief versus risk of infection. Discuss with patient and use clinical discretion.

Equipment

- 21G (green) needle and 20-mL syringe.
- Dressing towel and chlorhexidine skin preparation.
- Wound dressing.

Consent

- The main risk is infection (~1:1000 will become infected as a result of this procedure). Document consent in notes.
- A small amount of local anaesthetic can be used (e.g. 5 mL 1% lidocaine), although many do not require this.

Procedure

- The knee should be in ~15° of flexion.
- Palpate the bony landmarks – superior-lateral pole of patella, tibial tuberosities. Consider marking with a permanent marker.
- Wearing sterile gloves, clean the skin thoroughly twice. Drape if available. Re-palpate landmarks.
- To aspirate from the supra-patella pouch, aim to enter just inferior to the superior-lateral border of the patella, in the 'soft spot'. This allows access to the large supra-patella pouch, communicating with the knee.
- Lightly holding the patella between the finger and thumb, use your other hand to introduce the needle.
- Continue whilst aspirating backwards until the fluid is withdrawn. There should be little resistance and little pain.
- If fluid stops flowing, the needle may need to be gently manoeuvred forwards or backwards to free the soft tissue.
- To empty the syringe leave the needle in place, disconnect and then reconnect the syringe (or use a 3-way tap). For therapeutic relief, continue aspirating the knee until no further fluid can be withdrawn or drawing back on the needle is painful.
- Apply a sterile elastoplast, and a wool and crepe for comfort.

- Note the appearance of fluid:
  - frank pus strongly suggests infection;
  - turbid cloudy fluid is likely infection;
  - frank blood is a haemarthrosis, which suggests acute injury;
  - fat globules within the aspirate confirms the presence of a fractures;
  - clear, straw-coloured fluid suggests a non-infected effusion.

Post-procedure care

- Elevation, apply ice, and rest.
- If there is suspected infection, decant the first syringe full into a sterile container and send to microbiology. Phone and warn them, whatever the hour. During the day urgent microscopy results can be ready within an hour. During the night, the results can be expected by 08.00. Ensure someone is taking the sample to the laboratory urgently; don't leave it for 'routine' porter collection.
- The presence of organisms, pus cells, and white blood cells suggest infection, although their absence does not exclude infection. Urate crystals suggest gout.

Pitfalls

Who not to aspirate:

- Those with suspected prosthetic knee infections (this is best done in theatre).
- Those with overlying skin infections (e.g. cellulitis, which can introduce infection into a sterile knee).
- If suspecting infection post-arthroscopy, aspirate away from the portal sites, so as not to push infection through them.

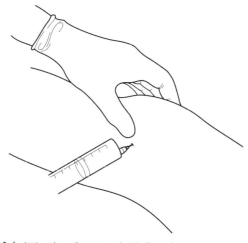

Fig. 9.3 Aspirating a knee. Approximately 15° of knee flexion, access the supra-patella pouch by entering inferiorly to the superiolateral pole of the patella.

⑦ Fractures in children

Fractures in children are common. Clinicians need to be aware of which injuries are simple versus those which are worrying. These include those which are likely to need surgery and those which may suggest non-accidental injury.

Common mechanisms of injury

- Mechanical falls are common in children, although a full history is still important to identify those who have passed out or are suffering from an occult medical problem (e.g. undiagnosed cardiac problems leading to collapse).
- The mechanism should match the injury. For example, a spiral humeral fracture would not be caused by walking into a door.

Clinical findings and examination

- Remember Advanced Trauma Life Support (ATLS) principles. Young children compensate for major injury well and don't necessarily tell you everything, e.g. they may have an occult splenic injury, which is only picked up by examining the abdomen.
- Pain, swelling, and deformity.
- The very young may not talk; they will be upset, hold the limb flexed, not move it, and be in pain when you touch it.

Common fractures

- Distal radial fractures.
- Radial/ulnar shaft fractures.
- Elbow fractures.
- Tibia/fibular fractures.
- Femoral fractures in infants.
- Pulled elbows.
- Finger and toe injuries.

Common types of fracture

- **Buckle fracture:** neither cortex break, but bend instead. Typically, minimally displaced. Surgery rarely needed.
- **Greenstick fracture:** one side of the cortex breaks, the other side bends. Typically, some deformity, ranging from mild to severe. Surgery depends on severity. See 📖 Distal radial fractures in children, p240, for example.
- **Growth plate injuries:** classified by Salter Harris, worsens as number increases (Fig. 9.4). Sometimes difficult to diagnose (especially V). Backslab these fractures, see in Fracture Clinic, or admit for ORIF if deformed. They need to be treated properly or growth arrest may occur.
- **Femoral fractures in toddlers:** femoral shaft fractures in children aged <4 years are typically transverse, and are displaced or non-displaced. They are well treated with traction. The legs are held elevated in a Gallows splint, where the hips are to 90° with the buttocks just off the bed; the body weight then acts as the traction force.

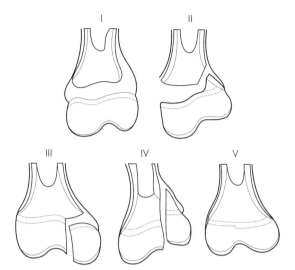

Fig. 9.4 Salter Harris classification of growth plate injuries. I Separation of the physis from the metaphysis; II Fracture through the physis and the metaphysis (most common); III Fracture through the epiphysis; IV Fracture through the physis, epiphysis, and metaphysis; V Crush injury to physis. Adapted from Bhangu & Keighley (2007). © Elsevier 2007.

Pathological fractures in children

A pathological fracture is caused by a fracture through an abnormal area of bone. In children, the following causes should be considered:
- Malignant tumours (e.g. osteoarcoma, Ewing's sarcoma).
- Benign tumours (bone cysts, osteochonromas).
- Osteomalacia (e.g. Ricket's disease).
- Osteogenesis imperfecta – multiple fractures at different stages of healing.

Signs of non-accidental injury

Have a high suspicion of index in order to protect children. Do not accuse the parents; admit, observe, investigate, and obtain senior paediatric opinion. Suspicious fractures include:
- Multiple fractures of different stages of healing.
- Injury not consistent with developmental age of child.
- Metaphyseal fractures.
- Posterior rib fractures.
- Spiral long bone fractures. Femoral fractures in infants <1-year-old (especially when spiral) are pathognomonic of NAI.
- Complex skull fractures.

Other signs include:
- Withdrawn, dejected child.
- Multiple bruises. Do not comment on the age of bruises, as they are so variable as to be unreliable.
- Inappropriate familiarity with unrelated adults.

General principles of management
- Be gentle and communicate well with children and parents.
- Backslab for pain and control. Children may not be compliant.
- Admit the obvious – open fractures, likely compartment syndromes, multiple injuries.
- Children with grossly deformed fractures (e.g. severely displaced distal radial fractures) should be admitted for MUA and then elevation.
- Stable fractures, such as distal radial fractures, which may or may not need surgery should be sent home in a backslab, starved that night, and discussed at the next morning's trauma meeting. If the child needs surgery, they can then come in immediately for the list, or be fed and brought back to Fracture Clinic if not.
- Children at risk or with uncertain home situations should be admitted.
- For more complex cases (e.g. medical problems, possible non-accidental injuries), children are better admitted under paediatricians with orthopaedic input. Otherwise, get a paediatric registrar review that day.
- Consent should be taken from a parent or, for older children, signed by them and countersigned by a parent. Mark limbs as for an adult.

Starving children
- For older children, starve as for adults.
- Younger children tolerate starvation less well. Thus, for morning lists (09.00 start), no solids from 03.00, but can have clear fluids until 06.00.

Reference
Bhangu, A., & Keighley, M. (2007) *The Flesh and Bones of Surgery*. Oxford: Elsevier.

ⓘ **Pathological fractures**

Pathological fractures are low energy fractures through abnormal bone, which has been weakened due to another disease process. These fractures, when the primary tumour is unknown, require thorough work-up prior to surgery (see Fig. 9.5).

Pathology
- Bony metastases are a common cause.
- Other causes including fibrous dysplasia, primary hyperparathyroidism, Paget's disease, multiple myeloma, bone cysts.
- Although osteoporosis technically causes pathological fractures (e.g. hip and Colles fractures), they are common and due to a widespread problem, rather than a specific local cause and, hence, are considered outside of this context.
- Cancers that commonly metastases to bone: breast, prostate (typically produce sclerotic lesions), thyroid, kidney, and lung.
- Common bones involved include the femur (especially hip), humerus (typically humeral shaft), vertebrae, and ribs (the last two do not necessarily require surgery and may be best admitted under medical specialities). However, any bone maybe affected.

History and examination
Typical suspicious findings, which should be considered when dealing with all fractures, are:
- Low energy injury, e.g. 'I was just getting up from of a chair'; 'I was walking along when my leg just gave way'.
- Look for recent weight loss, breast lumps, change in bowel habit, bone pain.
- Recent pain from the location suggesting development of metastases (above and beyond 'background' arthritic pain).
- Any history of cancer (current or previous).
- General examination: cachexia, anaemia, abdominal/breast/neck lumps. Digital rectal examination (DRE) to assess prostate.

Investigations
- Bloods: FBC, U&E, LFTs, calcium (vital), G&S. Tumour markers lack sensitivity and are not used in screening.
- X-ray: the X-ray shows a fracture through an abnormal lesion. Gain full length films of the bones involved (e.g. full length femur for hip fractures.
- Chest X-ray (primary and secondaries), mammograms for breast lumps, ultrasound abdomen/CT for abdominal lumps.
- CT chest/abdomen/pelvis is used to seek unknown primaries and stage known cancers.
- Bone scans assess for further metastases.
- Oncologists should be involved early.

Management

- Resuscitate with ABC. Correct lethal hypercalcaemia with fluids and IV bisphosphonates.
- Patients are investigated before surgical treatment; organize a bone scan, and a CT chest/abdomen/pelvis for unknown primaries.
- Admit and elevate/stabilize fractures. For fractures of the hip, bed rest is needed.
- **Prepare for theatre:** bloods, G&S, ECG, CXR.
- Ensure you communicate to the receiving team your suspicions.
- Surgical fixation options include IM nailing, arthroplasty, and occasionally plating. Bone is sent for histology (e.g. femoral head during hip hemiarthroplasty).
- Impending fractures can be prophylactically fixed, although this may not be suitable if life-expectancy is low. Any surgical fixation should be designed to outlive the patient.

Pitfalls

- Not suspecting pathological fractures through inadequate history and X-ray interpretation.
- Failing to get full length bone films, missing the true length of lesions and further lesions.

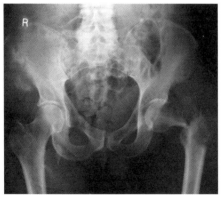

Fig. 9.5 There is a left proximal femur fracture, through a lytic lesion. There is further bony destruction in the right iliac crest. CXR and CT chest/abdomen/pelvis revealed a large left hilar mass, which was the primary.

:O: Post-operative bleeding

Post-operative bleeding is common following orthopaedic operations. Most is minor bleeding and non-problematic, although rarely continued bleeding from major joint arthroplasty (in particular the hip and knee) may become serious and life-threatening. Bleeding may occur from large vessels once a tourniquet has been released, especially soon after closure of the wound and application of dressings.

Presentation

- Bleeding can be immediately post-operative (e.g. in recovery), in the early post-operative period (e.g. first 24 h), or may be delayed and present with infected haematomas (late, 4–10 days).
- Bleeding may be indicated by high output into drains or oozing/soaked wound dressings.
- Signs of hypovolaemic shock (hypotension, tachycardia, confusion, pallor, and clamminess) are late signs and indicate dangerous blood loss.

Examination and investigations

- Examine wound and drains, and document volume of contents.
- Examine wound dressings. **Note:** if they are oozing and/or soaked in blood, do not remove any layers of the dressing now (see 📖 Post-operative bleeding, Initial measures to control post-operative bleeding, p162).
- Only basic investigation are needed. Blood pressure, pulse, oxygen saturations. Send blood for Hb and ensure a G&S is active.

Management

- Resuscitate with ABC.
- Ensure IV access if maintained and use IV fluids initially. Blood products may be needed if bleeding continues.

Initial measures to control post-operative bleeding

- Do not remove wound dressings. This will make bleeding worse by removing pressure. If wound dressings are oozing and soaked, apply further pressure dressings.
- Well localized direct pressure is the best place to start. For the knee, place folded gauze over existing dressings and wrap firmly with a new crepe. For the hip, apply folded gauze over existing dressings and apply firmly stretched Mepore® (or similar vapour-permeable adhesive film dressing) over the top (or wrap a crepe around the top of the thigh). Apply pressure with a gloved fist.
- If still oozing and the patient is shocked
  - elevate the limb and consider tilting the bed head down/feet up;
  - a tourniquet is useful. Get a pneumatic one from theatre and apply with appropriate padding.
- The patient may require blood products.
- If the patient continues to bleed, they may need to be taken back to theatre. Get senior surgeons and anaesthetists involved early.

- If bleeding settles, the patient can be monitored on the ward and repeat haemoglobin checked.
- Do not remove the drain until bleeding has settled. Ask the nurses to carefully document drain output.
- If bleeding is from the upper limb, elevate, and apply pressure dressings, although check the integrity of the distal pulses.
- If the patient continues to bleed, continue resuscitation, ask for senior help, keep NBM.

Pitfalls

- Removing haemostatic dressings to look at wounds.
- Under-estimating severity.
- Failing to elevate the upper limb post-operatively.

Pelvis

☠️ Types of pelvic fractures

Classifying pelvis fractures helps to describe and direct treatment, as well as being able to predict the likelihood of other injuries. As part of initial resuscitation, treat hypovolaemia, seek associated injuries and stabilize the pelvis with a commercial splint. Initial management of pelvic fractures is dealt with in 📖 Pelvic fractures, Management, p52.

Young and Burgess pelvic fracture classification (Fig. 10.1)

- Lateral compression (LC)
- Anterior-posterior compression (APC)
- Vertical shear (VS)
- Combination

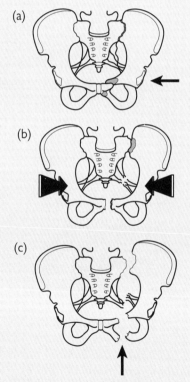

Fig. 10.1 (a) Lateral compression fracture. (b) Open book fracture – anterior-posterior compression. (c) Vertical sheer fracture.

Lateral compression fractures
- Most common type of pelvic fracture (see Fig. 10.2).
- Lateral compression fractures result in internal rotation of the affected hemi-pelvis, typically from side-on impacts in RTCs.
- Pelvic volume is reduced, so bleeding is less of a problem than associated head and intra-abdominal injuries.
- They range from simple to complex, multiple-traumatized (types I–III).

Anterior-posterior compression fractures
- The common feature of these injuries is disruption to the pubic symphysis, caused by the 'opening' nature of the anterior-posterior compression forces. Hence, these injuries are known as *open book fractures* (types I–III).
- When involving the posterior sacro-iliac joints, these are *rotationally unstable and vertically stable*. If there is no posterior component, these fractures may be stable (type I, symphysis separation <2.5 cm).
- *Pelvic volume is increased,* leading to a high rate of pelvic bleeding, with untamponaded haematomas expanding rapidly into the retroperitoneum. Exanguination may occur.
- There is a strong association with brain and intra-abdominal injury. Initial life-saving therapy is application of a sheet or SAM splint.

Vertical shear fractures
- These typically result from a fall from height.
- There is commonly ipsilateral pubic rami and sacro-iliac joint disruption due to shearing forces, rendering the fracture *rotationally unstable and vertically unstable.*

Thus, external fixation may be suitable for APC II/III, LC II/III, VS, and combination fractures.

Effect on pelvic volume

- **Lateral compression fractures:** reduced pelvic volume.
- **Open book fractures:** increased pelvic volume.

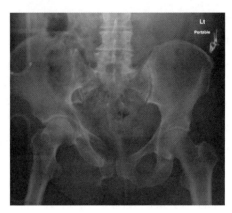

Fig. 10.2 AP pelvis of a right-sided lateral compression fracture. Note fractures through the pubic rami and ileum at the sacroiliac joint. Initial resuscitation required a chest drain for a pneumothorax.

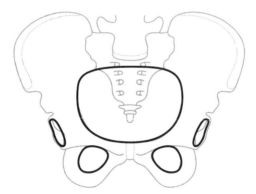

Fig. 10.3 The pelvis can be considered as a ring. A solid ring is difficult to break in only one place, and so always look for the second injury, either a smaller fracture or sacro-iliac disruption. Look for two fractures in a single ring; this then counts as one fracture in a bigger ring.

Other pelvic fractures

These fractures are typically rotationally and vertically stable. They are fractures either not involving the pelvic ring or, if involving the pelvic ring, are minimally displaced and, hence, stable. They are generally treated with bed rest for analgesia and then mobilization as pain allows.

Pubic rami fractures

Common in the elderly following falls. These are treated non-operatively with analgesia and mobilization as pain allows. May need referral to medical team/rehabilitation if unable to mobilize. Fracture Clinic follow-up is not required for simple fractures in the elderly. They can also occur in younger patients as the result of trauma, where initial management is the same, although follow-up is needed.

Avulsion fractures

- The result of muscle contraction avulsing bony fragments. Affect all ages, e.g. young athletes and the elderly. Patients who can mobilize are sent home. Management is conservative, although ORIF can be considered later for painful non-unions.
- **Typical muscles and associated fractures:**
  - anterior superior iliac spine and sartorius;
  - anterior inferior iliac spine and rectus femoris;
  - iliac crest and abdominal muscles.

Minimally displaced ring fractures

These are typically superior pubic rami fractures and iliac wing injuries. Minimal displacement requires only symptomatic treatment. Effective analgesia is provided by sitting on a rubber ring and avoiding constipation.

Coccyx fractures

- These occur after falling in a seated position onto a hard surface. Routine X-ray is not necessary as it does not change treatment. If needed, lateral X-rays show variable fracture patterns.
- Treatment is symptomatic. Effective analgesia is provided by sitting on a rubber ring and avoiding constipation. All are safely sent home with Fracture Clinic follow-up and only need orthopaedic review/admission if open. If painful non-union takes hold, excision can be performed.

Sacral fractures

- **Unstable fractures** are associated with high energy transfer, and are part of an unstable pelvic fracture pattern.
- **Simple transverse fractures** from low energy falls typically occur in the elderly, and are invariably non-displaced or minimally displaced. Treat symptomatically.
- **Sacral nerve roots** may be involved giving rise to lower limb neurological symptoms. These patients can be investigated with CT and MRI scans to assess stability and nerve root involvement. Most should be admitted for investigation.
- A short period of bed rest is followed by safe mobilization.

Lower limb

:⚙: **Hip dislocations and acetabular fractures**

Dislocations of the hip can occur in the elderly with total hip replacements or in younger patients following major trauma where they are commonly associated with acetabular fractures.

Traumatic hip dislocation

This typically occurs when direct force is transmitted along the femur:
* The leg is held flexed, adducted, and internally rotated, and appears shortened.
* **Test** dorsiflexion of the foot and sensation below the knee to assess sciatic nerve involvement pre-reduction.
* **Diagnosis** is confirmed on AP pelvis and lateral hip X-ray. Most are posterior dislocations and there may be an associated acetabular fracture. The whole femur should be imaged to look for patella and femoral shaft fractures.
* The dislocated hip should be reduced as soon as possible to restore integrity to the femoral head and prevent damage to the sciatic nerve.
* **Reduction** is normally in theatre under sedation.
* Standing above the patient, flex the hip and knee, and pull upwards to provide traction, thus reducing the hip. An assistant holds the pelvis down to stabilize.
* Failure here requires a GA with full relaxation. If this fails, open reduction is required.
* Recheck sciatic nerve function and obtain check X-rays.
* Apply a Thomas splint to maintain stability and immobilization if the hip remains unstable. Seek senior orthopaedic advice.
* These patients need to be admitted for further assessment and safe mobilization. Avascular necrosis is a long-term complication.

Acetabular fractures

These may be associated with a dislocated hip or other pelvic fracture (see Fig. 11.1):
* AP pelvis X-ray shows disruption of the acetabular wall or floor.
* Classification is complex. Fractures can be considered as either displaced or non-displaced, with/without comminution.
* Patients should be admitted for bed rest and further assessment. Skin traction is applied in ED with T&O teams.
* CT scan is necessary to assess fracture pattern and stability.
* Non-displaced, stable fractures can be treated conservatively.
* Displaced or unstable fractures need ORIF.
* Bed-rest and traction may be used for some fractures, under the direction of those with specialist knowledge.

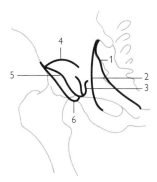

Fig. 11.1 Recognizing the acetabulum. 1 = ileopectineal line; 2 = ilioischial line; 3 = teardrop; 4 = floor of acetabulum; 5 = anterior wall; 6 = posterior wall.

Dislocated total hip replacement

The causes of dislocation include problems with the prosthesis and/or problems with the patient. Prosthetic components may have become loose or may have been sub-optimally positioned. Patient factors include poor compliance, poor musculature, and alcohol excess.

Presentation
- Dislocation of total hip replacements typically occurs in the elderly following a fall, twist, or low energy injury.
- The patient presents with pain and an inability to weight bear. On examination the limb is typically shortened.
- A pre-reduction neurovascular examination is important.

Investigations
- An AP pelvis radiograph diagnoses most.
- **Pre-operative assessment:** bloods, EGG, CXR.
- **Mark and consent:** consent must include the need for open reduction if closed fails (<5%).

Management
- Admit for reduction in theatre under an image intensifier.
- Techniques vary. Traction is applied on the pelvis by an assistant. With the knee flexed, flex the hip upwards, with internal and external rotation to reduce the hip.
- Check neurovascular status post-operatively.
- Follow with a brief period of bed rest in abduction (e.g. 24 h). Consider a Darby brace post-operatively to maintain reduction in selected elderly patients.
- Mobilize carefully with physiotherapists.
- If >2 dislocations, refer for hip revision surgery.

☼ Neck of femur fractures

'Hip' fractures are common in an increasingly elderly population. Patients with a neck of femur (NOF) fracture commonly present with co-existing multiple medical co-morbidities, both diagnosed and undiagnosed. These patients should be admitted from the ED as soon as possible (ASAP) onto a suitable ward and a more comfortable bed.

Pathology
- The majority are due to osteoporosis.
- Some are due to metastatic deposits (typically low energy).
- In the young, they are due to high energy impacts (e.g. RTC).

Presentation
- Most commonly follows a fall.
- **Useful questions:**
  - Why has the patient fallen? Can they remember tripping over the carpet? Do they remember events at all or did they black out and then fall? Did they have any pain in their chest or shortness of breath prior to the fall?
  - Did they bump their head when they fell or lose consciousness (remember subdural haematomas in the elderly)?
  - Did their leg 'just give way?' Did they hear a crack whilst getting out a chair? These are ultra-low mechanisms of injury, which suggest a pathological fracture. Ask about current and prior malignancies, and assess for weight loss and red flag symptoms.
  - What was their performance before the fracture? Were they walking to the shops on their own, pottering around the house of confined to a chair? Were they walking unaided/with stick/zimmer? Do they have existing arthritis of the hip (younger patients may benefit from total hip replacement)?
  - Note that some patients who have sustained minimally displaced, impacted stable fractures may be in pain, but have remained mobile.
- Assess medical co-morbidities, document, and prescribe all medications. If they haven't brought medications, ask someone to call in from the home with a list ASAP, or contact the care home or GP.
- What is the social situation? Do they live alone? Are they self-caring? How many carers a day?

Signs, symptoms, and clinical findings
- Pain over the hip and in the groin.
- The affected limb is often shortened and externally rotated. However, not all will be – with impacted, stable fractures, the limb may appear normal.
- Inability to straight leg raise.
- Check for sensation in the foot and adequate pulses.
- A full examination is mandatory – the chest for infections, the heart for murmurs, the abdomen for other pathology, assess hydration.
- Document pulse, temperature (severe hypothermia may occur in those lying on the floor for some time), blood pressure, oxygen saturations.

Investigations
- **Bloods:** FBC, U&E, group and save/cross-match depending on proposed operative procedures. Check creatinine kinase if the patient has been lying on the floor for a long time (consider rhabdomyolysis).
- **ECG:** to assess for causes of collapse (acute coronary syndrome/silent MI, arrhythmia) and pre-operative assessment.
- **Chest X-rays:** often needed in the presence of chest signs (and often part of the 'neck of femur pathway').
- **AP pelvis:** this must show at least the whole affected hip. Do not accept films that cut off the tip of the greater trochanter (you need to exclude trochanteric pull-off fractures).
- A lateral should be obtained.
- **Arterial blood gas:** should be performed for those with SaO_2 <95% on air to assist with pre-operative assessment.
- **The normal radiograph:** in most patients the fracture is obvious on radiographs. In some, radiographs may appear normal, but clinical suspicion is still high, especially those who were previously mobile. In these patients, a CT scan of the hip helps detect/exclude a hip fracture.

Management
- **Assess with ABC:** they may have sustained other injuries, and dehydration with hypothermia may be a complication of a prolonged period of waiting on the floor for someone to find them.
- **Give oxygen, IV rehydration, and analgesia:** these are basic resuscitative manoeuvres, which should be instigated in ED.
- **Analgesia:** e.g. 10 mg IV morphine titrated to pain relief.
- **IV fluids:** for initial resuscitation.
- Admit to the ward ASAP; consider pressure reduction beds (discuss with nursing staff who will assess using Waterlow score).
- Bed rest until theatre. Thus, prescribe prophylactic LMWH (e.g. enoxaparin 40 mg sc in the evening).
- **Consent:** if possible and if you know the procedure to be performed, obtain written consent now, as it prevents delays later and the family may be around now to help.
- Clearly mark the limb with a black permanent marker away from the hip (where the incision will be).
- A medical review (if needed) is often easier to get in the ED or Emergency Assessment areas before the patient goes to the ward.

:O: Types of neck of femur fracture

Although commonly termed as hip or NOF fractures, there are different types of fracture, which require different treatment. When discussing these fractures, start broadly, then move into more anatomically specific terminology. The broadest definition relates to fractures either side of the insertion of the joint capsule; intracapsular, and extra-capsular fractures.

The hip capsule

The capsule attaches just proximally to the intertrochanteric line. Fractures above this are intracapsular and below this are extracapsular. Since the major blood supply runs through the capsule, displaced intracapsular fractures cause capsular disruption and, therefore, have a high risk of avascular necrosis. Further sub-classification is possible (see Fig. 11.2):

- **Intracapsular fractures:** can be subcapital (below the head, I) or transcervical (across the neck, II).
- **Extracapsular fractures:** can be intertrochanteric (between the greater and lesser trochanters, III) or subtrochanteric (below the inter-trochanteric line, IV).

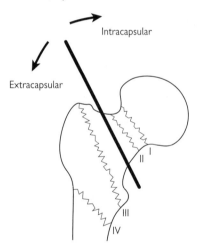

Fig. 11.2 Intra- and extracapsular fractures. Adapted from Bhangu and Keighley (2007). © Elsevier 2007.

Managing intracapsular fractures

- If these fractures are displaced, they are likely to disrupt the capsular blood supply to the femoral head, and so replacement of the displaced femoral head is needed (i.e. hemiarthroplasty). If patients had pre-existing arthritis in the hip and were fairly mobile, they may benefit from total hip replacement.
- If these fractures are non-displaced, preserve the patient's own femoral head (giving a better functional outcome) as the capsular blood supply

is unlikely to be disrupted. Commonly fixation with percutaneous screws or in some units dynamic hip screws can be used depending on consultant policy.

- Garden's classification helps define non displaced and displaced fractures and is based on the interpretation of the trabecular pattern in the antero-posterior X-ray (Fig. 11.3):
  - *non-displaced-* I is an incomplete fracture and II is complete but non-displaced
  - *displaced* - III is complete and partially displaced [trabeculae inline] and IV is completely displaced [trabeculae disrupted] fractures (Fig. 11.4).

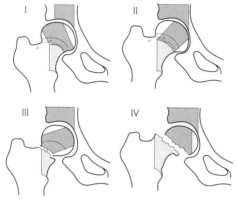

Fig. 11.3 Garden's classification of intracapsular fractures. I Non-displaced, incomplete; II Non-displaced, complete; III Complete partially displaced; IV Completely displaced. Adapted from Bhangu and Keighley (2007). ©Elsevier 2007.

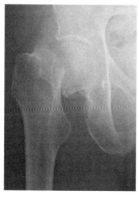

Fig. 11.4 Displaced intracapsular NOF fracture. The patient was admitted for a hip hemiarthoplasty.

Managing extracapsular fractures

- These fractures do not interfere with the femoral head capsular blood supply and the fracture should be reduced and fixed.
- For intratrochanteric fractures a dynamic hip screw (DHS) fixes the fracture and permits some movement to allow the natural impaction that takes place during healing (Fig. 11.5).
- Subtrochanteric fractures may be too low for a DHS, and so a proximal femoral nail may be needed.

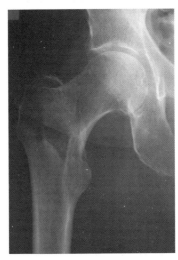

Fig. 11.5 An extracapsular NOF fracture, suitable for a dynamic hip screw.

Hip fractures in the young

- These are often the result of high impact trauma in patients <50 years, and may be associated with other serious injuries. These patients should be received in Resuscitation with a Trauma team.
- Look for associated acetabular and other pelvic fractures.
- When intracapsular, these are orthopaedic emergencies. The need to preserve the young patient's femoral head is paramount and so surgical fixation should be carried out as soon as possible.
- For extracapsular fractures, there is more time to plan since the femoral head is not at risk.

For young patients with intracapsular hip fractures (typically young trauma patients), inform seniors immediately, no matter the hour. Theatre is needed as soon as possible to preserve the femoral head.

Not for theatre
- Some elderly patients with a NOF fracture will be judged by seniors to be too unwell to tolerate either a general or spinal anaesthetic. These patients have a high mortality and most do not leave hospital alive.
- They should be given adequate fluids to relieve dehydration, analgesia to relieve pain, and oxygen to relieve breathlessness. A review by the medical registrar early is vital (i.e. in ED). The resuscitation status may need to be discussed with seniors, patients, and family/next of kin.
- With bed rest, medical reviews, and nursing care, some patients may improve enough to be taken to theatre or for subsequent transfer to a nursing home.

Reference
Bhangu A. and Keighley, M. (2007) *The Flesh and Bones of Surgery*. Oxford: Elsevier.

:☼: **Lower femoral fractures**

Supracondylar fractures

- These occur in children and adults.
- Check for neurovascular deficit.
- In children, non-displaced fractures can be treated in plaster cast.
- In adults, rotation often occurs, which leads to displacement and so ORIF is needed. Some non-displaced fractures may be treatable in plaster.
- Admit patients needing ORIF for analgesia and temporary plaster of Paris (PoP) backslab.

These may be displaced or non-displaced, and may be comminuted. Non-displaced fractures may be treatable by plaster, although many advocate early surgical fixation. Displaced and intra-articular fractures need to be admitted for ORIF. Consider skin traction.

⊙ Injuries to the patella

Fracture to the patella

Presentation

The patella is typically fractured either after a direct blow (e.g. fall onto the knee) or as an avulsion fracture after strong muscular contraction.

Signs, symptoms, and clinical findings

- The patient is in pain over the patella, and cannot raise a straight leg OR extend the knee (the extensor mechanism of the lower limb is lost as the 'anchoring' functions of the patella are lost).
- A palpable gap is often felt at the level of the fracture or at the superior/inferior poles of the patella in cases of avulsion fractures.

Investigations

- AP and lateral X-rays of the patella are needed.
- Bipartate patellae are reasonably common and may look like a fracture on X-ray. This is a congenital variant where a small fragment of the patella is not attached to the rest, typically in the upper outer quadrant. The bone piece is rounded at its edges in contrast. Fractures have sharp edges.
- Patella fracture patterns include vertical, non-displaced horizontal, displaced horizontal, and comminuted.

Management

- Hold in a cylinder cast for comfort if going home.
- Vertical and undisplaced horizontal fracture can be treated in a cylinder plaster cast for 6 weeks, with check X-rays.
- Displaced horizontal fractures often require ORIF. Admit with an above-knee backslab.
- Very comminuted fractures may be best treated with excision (admit).
- Otherwise, if patient is safe for home and does not live alone, they can be discharged.

Dislocation of the patella

- This typically occurs in young females as a congenital anomaly, or as the result of direct trauma in others.
- The patella typically dislocates laterally.
- The patient may present with the patella dislocated or after it has spontaneously reduced. This may be first or recurrent dislocation.
- Reduce by pushing the patella medially, whilst extending the knee. Provide Entonox® for analgesia.
- Treat first dislocations in a cylinder plaster cast for 3 weeks, followed by physiotherapy.
- Patients can go home, partial weight-bearing (PWB) with crutches, with Fracture Clinic review.

☼ Dislocation of the knee

This is a significant injury, although they may occur from high or low energy mechanism.

There are five potential directions of dislocation, with anterior and posterior being the most common:

- **Anterior:** the tibia is dislocated anteriorly due to severe hyperextension.
- **Posterior:** direct injuries to the front of the tibia (anterior-posterior force).
- **Medial/lateral/rotatory:** less common.

Check presence of **distal foot pulses**. The popliteal pulse is (a) difficult to feel in these injuries and (b) the injury is quite often at the level of the trifurcation.

The knee should be reduced ASAP. Give Entonox® for initial pain relief and titrated IV morphine in Resuscitation. For anterior dislocations, provide traction down the leg and gently push back on the tibial head (thus reducing anterior dislocations). Posterior dislocations are reduced by pulling the tibia forwards.

Always check neurovascular deficit both *before* and *after* any reduction procedure.

- **Treat in a loose above knee backslab and admit.** Regular checks must be made on distal (foot) pulses overnight.
- Once pain has settled, clinical assessment, and MRI scans assess the state of the ligaments of the knee. Depending on results, surgical or non-surgical management can be used.

Indications for acute surgical intervention

- Failure of closed reduction.
- Persistent absence of distal foot pulses mandate an urgent vascular opinion and surgical exploration.

⊙ Ligamental and meniscal injuries

These injuries are common in sports people, but also occur in older, less active patients. They can be extremely painful even in the absence of fracture.

Ligamentous injuries

Presentation

The patient reports a twisting injury or that their 'foot got caught in the ground' whilst running.

Signs, symptoms, and clinical findings
- They frequently describe a popping sensation, a cracking sound, immediate pain, and/or immediate swelling. They may or may not have been able to bear weight.
- An effusion forms. This may be undetectable, mild or tense and painful.
- The knee should be fully examined to detect fractures, joint line tenderness and ligamentous instability. Some patients may be in too much pain to tolerate full examination at present.

Investigations

AP and lateral views of the knee exclude fractures and identify smaller avulsion fractures.

Types of injury
- **Anterior cruciate ligament:** anterior drawer sign positive. Often associated with medial collateral ligament or medial meniscal injuries. Look carefully for tibial spine fractures.
- **Posterior cruciate ligament:** posterior drawer sign is positive. Often not injured in isolation, look for medial/lateral collateral injuries.
- **Lateral collateral ligament:** look for a fracture of the fibula head.
- **Medial collateral ligament:** due to a valgus stress. Associated with medial meniscal and ACL injuries (the 'unhappy triad').

Management

- Analgesia and elevation.
- For minor injuries where the pain is minimal and the patient can weight bear, they can be mobilized fully weight bearing (FWB) and sent home. A strapping (e.g. Robert Jones bandage) may help. Follow-up should be arranged, although a definitive diagnosis may never be reached and may not be necessary.
- For those with more significant injuries who are in pain, a cricket pad splint/modified Roberts Jones bandage or above-knee backslab provide comfort and stability. These patients should be given crutches and made non-weight bearing (NWB) until clinic.
- Some patients will be in too much pain or cannot tolerate crutches – they may need admission until pain settles.
- Very tense haemarthrosis may need aspiration (see 📖 Aspirating the knee, p154), although the risks of infection should be discussed. Adequate drainage relieves pain and allows re-examination.
- Undisplaced tibial spine fractures with ACL ruptures are treated acutely with an above knee backslab, which can be converted later to a cylinder cast for a total of 6 weeks. Displaced tibial spine fractures require surgical fixation.
- MRI and arthroscopy can be discussed in Fracture Clinic.

Meniscal injuries

Presentation

- These are the result of twisting injuries, often with the knee flexed and typically in men.
- There is often a history of giving way after the injury.

Signs, symptoms, and clinical findings

- The patient is in pain and has difficulty weight bearing.
- The knee may be 'locked' – this is when the patient cannot fully extend the knee (they have typically lost the last 10–15° of full extension.
- An effusion may be present.
- Joint line tenderness is often present and McMurray's test may be positive.

Investigations

AP and lateral X-rays are needed to exclude fractures.

Management

- These patients can go home with a knee strapping +/– crutches for support. Fracture Clinic follow-up should be arranged.
- Depending on the patient and progress, an MRI scan may be needed.
- Those unable to mobilize may need to be admitted from ED probably for MRI scan and +/– early arthroscopy.
- Those with locked knees require admission (for analgesia, further assessment and possibly in-patient arthroscopy).

! **Tibial plateau fractures**

There is a lateral and medial tibial plateau, and although the majority of fractures are lateral, fractures involving both plateaus, as well as the ligamentous complex of the knee occur.

Presentation

Typically follow falls, although mechanisms vary.

Signs, symptoms, and clinical findings

- The knee is painful and swollen.
- Very tense effusions represent haemarthroses.
- The patient cannot weight bear and may not be able to tolerate examination of the ligaments of the knee.
- Test distal neurovascular status. If the fibula head is fractured, check for foot drop.

Investigations

- AP and lateral X-rays of the knee. Ensure that you can see to the bottom of the fracture, tibial films may be needed.
- Look for the tibial plateau fractures (Fig. 11.7), as well as fibula head fractures.
- Fractures are classified according to Schatzker (Fig. 11.6), where 6 is the worst type of injury.
- Stress radiographs may be needed later to test for stability.
- Complex fractures often require CT scans to assess configuration.

Management

- Admit.
- Place in an above-knee backslab for stability and analgesia.
- Consider aspiration only for very tense, painful haemarthrosis.
- Discuss with seniors and book CT scan once admitted if needed.
- Undisplaced fractures may be managed non-operatively in a plaster backslab and with crutches.
- Prepare for theatre. Mark, bloods, ECG +/− consent when decision to operate is made.

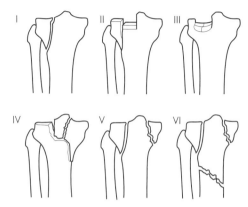

Fig. 11.6 Schatzker classification of tibial plateau fractures. I Wedge fracture of tibial plane (most common); II Wedge fracture and depression of the lateral plateau; III No fracture, lateral plateau depressed; IV Wedge fracture of the medial tibial plane; V With a diaphysis or metaphysic fracture; VI Bicondylar wedge fractures of both plateaux. Adapted from Bhangu and Keighley (2007). © Elsevier 2007.

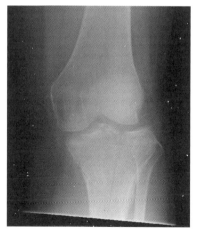

Fig. 11.7 Tibial plateau fracture. Note that the fracture extends down the tibial shaft. Another X-ray was required to assess how far it extends.

Reference

Bhangu A. and Keighley, M. (2007)*The Flesh and Bones of Surgery*. Oxford: Elsevier.

ⓘ **Tibia and fibula shaft fractures**

These bones are commonly injured following twisting forces or direct blows to the leg. As with the ankle, the incidence of open fractures is relatively high.

Presentation

Any mechanism that places stresses on the lower limb – sports injuries, falls, direct blows, RTCs, etc.

Signs, symptoms, and clinical findings

- There is pain, swelling, deformity, and inability to weight bear.
- The fracture fragments may displace and tent the skin, necessitating prompt reduction.
- If the skin is pierced, the fracture is open. With footballers and sports players, the wound may be dirty with grass and mud.
- Assess the calf for evidence of compartment syndrome.

Investigations

- AP/lateral X-rays of the whole tibia/fibula, to include the ankle.
- Fractures may be transverse, spiral, or comminuted (Fig. 11.8).
- Fractures in children may be greenstick or complete.

Management

- Treat open fractures as such.
- Call seniors early if evidence of *compartment syndrome* and release any backslab or dressing.
- **Low energy:**
  - *Undisplaced, simple fractures* – treated in an above-knee backslab.
  - *Minimally displaced stable fractures* – treated with manipulation and plaster cast. Consider admission for analgesia/observation.
- **High energy:**
  - They are nearly always admitted for elevation and observation for compartment syndrome.
  - *Spiral fractures* – even when minimally displaced, are potentially unstable. They can be treated conservatively if non-displaced, but require weekly monitoring.
  - *Displaced, unstable fractures* – e.g. spiral displaced fractures, are treated best treated with surgical fixation (e.g. intramedullary nailing, plate and screws, ex-fix). Admit.
  - *Fragmented, comminuted fractures* – difficult to treat. These patients should be admitted; ex-fix may be needed.
- **Children:**
  - minimally displaced angulation can be accepted and the child treated in an above knee plaster cast;
  - angulated fractures should be reduced under GA;
  - off-ended/very displaced fractures may require surgical fixation.

Who to send home/who to admit

Most are admitted for elevation and observation for compartment syndrome (especially high energy injuries). Those with undisplaced simple fractures, soft compartments, and minimal pain can go home with an above-knee backslab and crutches, to come back to the next Fracture Clinic.

Pitfalls

- Failing to assess for compartment syndrome.
- Sending home patients with significant fractures who need to be admitted for elevation/monitoring of compartment syndrome.

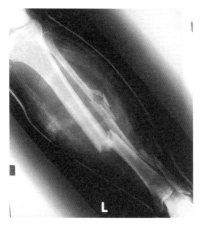

Fig. 11.8 Closed tibial and comminuted segmented fibular fracture. The patient was admitted and placed in a backslab.

Isolated fibular fractures

- An isolated fibular fracture can be treated symptomatically, with a below-knee walking plaster cast.
- However, the full tibia and fibula must be X-rayed to assess for a second injury (e.g. ankle fracture).
- Assess for common peroneal nerve damage with fibular neck fractures (foot drop).
- The presence of a second ipsilateral fibular fracture may require surgical fixation. Discuss with someone senior.
- A *Maisonneuve fracture* typically involves a fibular neck fracture and a medial malleolar fracture. The interosseous membrane is torn up to the level of the fibular fracture and, therefore, renders the syndosmosis unstable. Most of these patients require theatre, although may be sent home and seen in the Fracture Clinic if analgesia controlled. These patients should be placed in a backslab.

ⓘ **Ankle fractures**

Ankle fractures are common and affect all ages. Patients can be broadly thought of as those requiring theatre, those not requiring theatre, and those who may need theatre if plaster fails. Either way, open fractures and closed swelling are issues in these patients.

Presentation

Most commonly follows a fall. Try and establish whether it was an inversion or eversion type injury.

Signs, symptoms, and clinical findings

- Pain, swelling, tenderness, inability to weight bear (see 📖 Ankle fractures, Ottawa rules, p190).
- Look for open fractures. Due to proximity of the skin to the bone, open fractures in this region are common. Bone may either protrude or a small puncture wound may be visible (from 'in-out' movement of the bone).
- Check and document distal pulses and sensation.

Ottawa rules

The **Ottawa rules** help determine who needs an ankle X-ray (Fig. 11.9). They are extremely sensitive and reduce the need for unnecessary X-rays. If any of the following are present, ankle X-rays are indicated:

- Tenderness around the posterior edge of the medial or lateral malleolus and to 6 cm above.
- Tenderness over the navicular (needs a foot X-ray).
- Tenderness over the base of 5th metatarsal (needs a foot X-ray).
- Inability to weight bear 4 steps *both* immediately and in the ED.

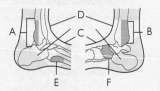

Fig. 11.9 A. Posterior edge or tip of lateral malleous, 6 cm; B. Posterior edge or tip of medial lateral malleous, 6 cm; C. Mid-foot zone; D. Malleolar zone; E. Base of fifth metatarsal; F. Navicular. Adapted from Stiel, I et al. BMJ 1995; 311: 594–597.

Investigations

- **AP and lateral ankle views:** if in doubt obtain full length tibia/fibula films.
- **Assess for talar shift.** the distance between the tibial and talar articular surfaces should be the same as from the talus to medial malleolus (Fig. 11.11).

Weber's classification of ankle fractures

This relates the fibular fracture to the syndesmosis (the ligamentous attachment between the tibia and fibula), which also guides management (Fig. 11.10):
- **Weber A:** the fibular fracture is below the syndesmosis. They are avulsion fractures found below the mortise (joint line) and are stable, thus commonly only require a PoP.
- **Weber B:** the fibular fracture is at the level of the syndesmosis. They are spiral fibular fractures that start at the level of the mortise and may or may not involve the syndesmosis. Thus, these fractures may be stable or unstable. If signs of instability fix with ORIF. Otherwise treat in PoP and monitor in Fracture Clinic.
- **Weber C:** the fibular fracture is above the syndesmosis. They disrupt the syndesmosis and interosseous ligaments, and are thus unstable. Admit for elevation and ORIF.

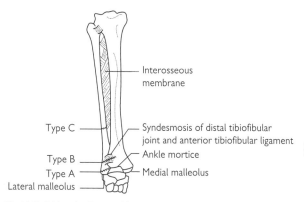

Interosseous membrane

Type C

Syndesmosis of distal tibiofibular joint and anterior tibiofibular ligament

Ankle mortice

Type B

Type A

Medial malleolus

Lateral malleolus

Fig. 11.10 Weber classification of fractures around the ankle. The higher the fracture, the more likely surgical fixation is needed. Adapted from Bhangu and Keighley (2007). © Elsevier 2007.

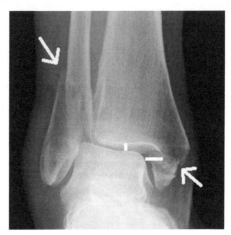

Fig. 11.11 Bilateral malleolar Weber B fracture. Both medial and lateral malleoli are fractured (arrows). The fibula component is at the level of the syndesmosis. There is marked talar shift, indicated by the difference in length of the solid white lines. This fracture configuration is unstable, and the patient was admitted for elevation and subsequent ORIF.

Management

- Open fractures require formal debridement in theatre.
- **Weber A or B,** and likely stable, place in a backslab, give instructions for elevation and send home NWB with Fracture Clinic FU.
- **Weber C or obviously unstable**, admit for elevation and ORIF. Place in a backslab for comfort and mould to correct major deformities, elevate and treat with icepacks.
- Many **bimalleolar** (medial and lateral malleoli) and **trimalleolar** (medial, lateral, and posterior malleoli) are unstable and require ORIF.
- In children, fractures in this region commonly affect the growth plate and so are Salter-Harris fractures (see 📖 Fractures in children, p156).
- Small, minimally displaced *avulsion fractures* can be treated symptomatically, although are commonly managed in an air cast boot.
- Swelling is an important pre-operative issue. Gross swelling prevents ORIF as the skin will not close well. Thus, if swollen, time may be needed until this subsides (this may take up to 2 weeks). To reduce swelling, immobilize in a loose backslab, elevate on a frame (or 2 pillows), apply ice (wrapped in a protective layer), and advise bed rest.

Who to send home

- Most with simple fractures not requiring surgery (Weber's A and stable Weber's B) can go home in a backslab and be brought back to next Fracture Clinic.
- Patients needing surgery (Weber's C, unstable Weber's B, bimalleolar/ trimalleolar fractures) should be admitted for ice and elevation, and to get onto the next available list (unless a clear plan for non-swollen patients is made during admission from Fracture Clinic onto a certain list).

Pilon fracture

Also known as tibial Plafond fractures, these are complex injuries caused by high energy vertical compression forces. The talus is driven upwards into the tibia. Occasionally, they occur following low energy injuries in skiers:

- Fracture pattern includes intra-articular ankle fracture with a tibial metaphyseal fracture. Other components include fractures of the medial malleolus and/or fibula.
- Soft tissue damage is often extensive, and the risk of open fracture is high. Check distal pulses – if absent seek vascular opinion.
- The lumbar spine should be checked for associated lumbar compression fracture.
- Placed in a loose backslab and admit for elevation.
- All fractures require a CT scan.
- ORIF is required for these complex fractures. Open fractures are treated as such, although definitive surgical fixation can be delayed.

References

Bhangu A. and Keighley, M. (2007) *The Flesh and Bones of Surgery*. Oxford: Elsevier.

Stiel, I., *et al.* (1995) Multicentre trial to introduce the Ottawa ankle rules for use of radiography in acute ankle injuries. *Br Med J* **311:** 594–7.

☼ Ankle dislocation

Dislocation of the ankle is an orthopaedic emergency and is always associated with an ankle fracture. With little soft tissue to compensate for the dislocation, skin is rapidly placed under tension, and the arteries to the foot are rapidly compressed (as opposed to other large joints, such as the shoulder). Ischaemia will occur rapidly unless the ankle is reduced.

- Most follow a serious traumatic injury (e.g. heavy fall or direct blow) and concurrent fracture is common.
- The joint is markedly displaced in some; the foot is cold, pale, and pulses are impalpable. Hence, this is a clinical diagnosis.
- **Reduction should be performed before X-rays.** Give adequate analgesia (Entonox® or morphine) first, and consider sedation with midazolam by an experienced practitioner e.g. ED Registrar/Consultant in the Resus room with full monitoring.
- One hand holds the ankle, the other the calf; a second person can provide traction from the knee. Provide downwards traction via the heel and slide the ankle back into place. You may have to exaggerate the deformity first. When the ankle reduces, pain resolves, the foot becomes pink, and pulses are restored.
- Hold in a backslab immediately, and gain AP and lateral X-rays.
- Admit for elevation and further Orthopaedic management.

① Calcaneal fractures

Calcaneal fractures follow falls from height onto the heels, and are associated with other lower limb fractures, and spinal fractures, due to transmitted forces from the impact (Fig. 11.12).

Presentation
- Fall from height onto heels.
- Bear in mind that a fall may be a suicide attempt.

Signs, symptoms, and clinical findings
- Swelling, bruising, lateral tilt.
- Assess swelling: compartment syndrome of the foot may occur.
- Assess the contralateral heel for bilateral fracture.
- Assess the ipsilateral knee, hip, and pelvis for fracture.
- Assess the lumbar and thoracic spine for tenderness, suggestive of associated fracture.

Investigations
- AP and lateral calcaneus X-rays are needed.
- AP and lateral of the lumbar spine if in doubt (also for knee, pelvis, and thoracic spine dependent on clinical findings).
- **Bohler's salient angle:** this traditionally provided a radiological guide as to who may need surgery. However, now all patients have a CT scan alongside significant orthopaedic and radiological consultation, and so decisions are no longer made based upon this. Draw a line through the anterior articular process through the posterior articular surface. Draw a second line through the superior angle of the tuberosity through the posterior articular surface. The angle between these two lines is normally around 40°. An angle of <20° suggests calcaneal fracture, as the heel 'flattens;' ORIF may be needed.

Management
- Assess with ATLS.
- **Admit** to allow swelling to subside and for CT scan.
- Swelling can become severe in the coming hours/days, and so admission with elevation and ice are recommended. A loose backslab can help the pain, although elevation on pillows or Braun frame is better if swelling is likely to continue.
- CT scan is required to assess fracture pattern (there are 7 types) and involvement of the sub-talar joint.
- Depending on the patient's status and CT finding, these fractures can be managed surgically or conservatively.

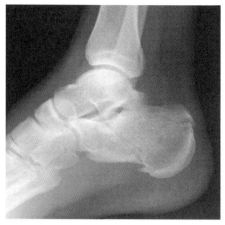

Fig. 11.12 This patient with a calcaneal fracture was admitted for elevation. Swelling became gross the next day. A CT scan with 3D reconstruction was obtained.

ⓘ Foot fractures

Fractures to the foot are common. Toe fractures are often crush or open injuries. Do not forget to assess for swelling, as compartment syndrome complicates some more significant fractures.

Presentation

Fall, awkward step (twisting and traction forces), dropping something, getting the foot caught.

Signs, symptoms, and clinical findings

- Swelling and bruising are common. Assess for compartment syndrome. Assess the ankle for involvement.
- Degloving injuries (with or without fracture) need urgent plastic surgery review. Early referral to a trauma centre may be needed.

Investigations

AP and lateral/oblique X-rays. Try and suggest which bones are involved so that the radiographer can give the best views.

Hind/mid-foot fractures and their management

- **Lisfranc injuries:** the Lisfranc joint is where the metatarsals meet the tarsal bones; they are connected by the tough Lisfranc ligament. Lisfranc tarsometatarsal fracture – dislocation injuries are fracture-dislocations to these joints and there are many patterns. Radiographically suspect with multiple fractures, malaligned metatarsals/tarsals, malaligned metatarsal shafts. Request a 'true lateral' X-ray. Swelling is profuse with significant injuries; admit all for elevation and monitoring for compartment syndrome (Fig. 11.13).
  - apply a below knee backslab, then open the front until comfortable (hence, forming a 'gutter splint');
  - a CT scan is needed;
  - stress testing under GA guides ORIF; isolated dislocations without fractures often require k-wire stabilization.
- **Dislocation of the talus:** due to a severe inversion injury, requires prompt reduction under GA.

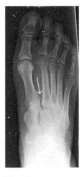

Fig. 11.13 Lisfranc fracture – dislocation.

Metatarsal fractures and their management

- **Base of 5ᵗʰ metatarsal:** most common fracture of the lower limb (Fig. 11.14). Typically, an avulsion fracture after inversion strain due to attachment of peroneous brevis. Non-displaced or moderately displaced fractures are treated with a crepe support for 2–3 weeks if moderate pain or walking cast for ~6 weeks if pain is more marked.
- **Jones fracture:** a base of 5th metatarsal fracture distal to the intermetatarsal joint (1–2 cm distal to the proximal tip). It is caused by repeated stresses (e.g. young athletes). Treat in a below-knee NWB cast for 6–7 weeks. Consider internal fixation in professional athletes.
- **Dancer's fracture:** spiral fracture of the 5th metatarsal neck (e.g. spiral movements in ballet dancers). AP, lateral, and oblique views are needed. Mildly displaced fractures are treated in a below knee cast for ~6 weeks. Displaced fractures require ORIF (admit of via clinic).
- **Undisplaced, shaft/neck fractures metatarsal 1–4:** often resulting from crush injuries, may be single or multiple. Undisplaced neck fractures can be treated conservatively (e.g. walking cast) and seen in Fracture Clinic.
- **Displaced, multiple fractures of metatarsals 1–4:** these result from significant crush injuries where lateral drift may be seen. Admit due to swelling and the need for surgical reduction. Manipulation +/– K-wires are used.

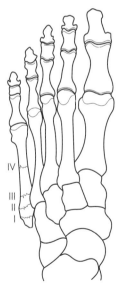

Fig. 11.14 5th metatarsal fractures. I Avulsion fracture; II Jones fracture; III Stress fracture; IV Mid-shaft transverse fracture.

Toe fractures and their management: toes

General

- Simple clinical toe fractures do not require an X-ray if there is no clinical deformity (except for big toe). Treat as a fracture, neighbour strap and advise the patient it will take up to 6 weeks to recover. No routine follow-up is required.
- Assess circulation with capillary refill. If swelling is compromising blood flow to the distal toe, admit for elevation and ice.
- Reduce deformities under digital block +/− Entonox®.
- Open fractures (e.g. open crush injuries) are admitted and treated as such. IV antibiotics and tetanus are given, and wounds may need to be debrided and closed in theatre.
- If the toe nail has been avulsed, the nail bed will need repair if damaged.
- **Big toe fractures:** often the result of heavy crush injuries; often open. Debride and close open wounds. Remove toe nail if necessary.
  If closed, neighbour strap and dress, with a walking toe platform for 4 weeks.

ⓘ Achilles tendon rupture

Trauma on-calls will attract other injuries to the lower limb, which do not involve fractures. Achilles tendon rupture is a lower limb tendon problem that presents to orthopaedics not infrequently.

Presentation
- Typically follows sudden muscular contraction (e.g. jumping, pushing off).
- Patient often reports the feeling of being kicked in the back of the leg, although without any contact or the patient actually hears a crack as the tendon ruptures.

Signs, symptoms, and clinical findings
- There is pain, swelling, poor walking, inability to stand on toes, a visible gap may be palpable in the tendon.
- **Simmond's test:** with the patient resting on their front, normally squeezing the calf contracts the muscles and causes a flinch of plantarflexion. Rupture of the tendon means this is lost and squeezing the tendon causes no reaction (Fig. 11.15).

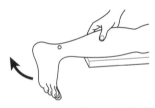

Fig. 11.15 Simmonds' test. Adapted from Bhangu & Keighley (2007).

Investigations
- A plain X-ray of the ankle reveals any associated avulsion fracture and a soft tissue gap at the level of the rupture may be visible.
- An ultrasound scan can define the extent of the injury if the diagnosis is in clinical question.

Management
- The patient should be placed in a plantar flexed cast, which approximates the ruptured tendon ends, and made NWB.
- The options for management are surgical or non-surgical.
- Young patients with high functional requirements (e.g. athletes) are good candidates for surgical repair. This affords lower re-rupture rates, although is associated with a risk of wound breakdown.

- The elderly or those with minimally displaced ruptures may be suitable for non-operative treatment, which usually involves a short period in a plaster cast, followed by an AFO with wedges and subsequently physiotherapy.
- The patient doesn't have to decide now. Bring back to the next Fracture Clinic for further discussion with seniors.
- Those presenting with re-ruptures are treated in the same way, although the need for surgical intervention is more likely.

Reference

Bhangu A. and Keighley, M. (2007) *The Flesh and Bones of Surgery*. Oxford: Elsevier.

⚠ **Quadriceps tendon rupture**

This is a rupture of the quadriceps tendon superior to the patella and is more common in men aged 60–70 years. There are many associated medical conditions, including hyperparathyroidism, diabetes, renal failure, arthritis, steroid use, gout.

Presentation

Typically follows strong contraction of the quadriceps muscle.

Signs, symptoms, and clinical findings

- It is associated with intense pain +/– haemarthrosis.
- The patella often 'sags' to sit inferiorly. Compare with the other side.
- There is loss of knee extension, and so a *straight leg raise* is impossible. Walking is not possible because of this.
- A gap superior to the patella may be palpable.

Investigations

A plain X-ray of the knee may show an inferiorly sitting patella.

Management

- Admit for early open repair (i.e. within 48 h).
- An above knee backslab can be applied for pain relief.
- Mark and consent for surgical repair.

① **Pretibial lacerations**

The skin over the tibia is thin, and often fragile and friable in the elderly. This is especially so in those on warfarin or steroids. Pretibial lacerations occur when the skin over the tibia is broken or torn, often due to a fall or direct trauma, usually without underlying bony injury. A haematoma accompanies the laceration, which may prevent closure of the skin.

Presentation
- Typically follows fall.
- Wounds may be clean or dirty.

Investigations
A plain X-ray excludes underlying bony injuries and may identify foreign bodies.

Management
Wounds should be cleaned. Check tetanus status. If the patient is unsure and the wound contaminated, treat with tetanus vaccine and immunoglobulin.

Closing pre-tibial lacerations

Simple wounds with little skin separation are best closed with sterile skin closure strips (e.g. Steri-strip®) in the ED (Fig. 11.16). **Do not** suture these wounds – the skin is fragile and friable, and may necrose if sutured:
- Dress in a crepe bandage and send home. Follow-up with the district nurse or a suitable clinic (A&E review, Plastics, or Fracture Clinic) should be arranged within a week.
- Heavily contaminated wounds (e.g. soil, debris) should be cleaned in ED and admitted for formal debridement in theatre. Give tetanus cover. Dress appropriately [e.g. a non-adherent dressing, such as paraffin gauze dressing (Jelonet®) (do not use a dry dressing)] and elevate.
- Those with significant skin loss, large underlying haematomas or marked skin separation should be admitted for assessment for surgery. The wound should still be initially cleaned and dressed in ED. Plastic surgery input is often required.
- Large haematomas are debrided in theatre with plastic surgery input; 'second look' surgery with split skin grafts covers significant skin loss.
- Mark and consent.

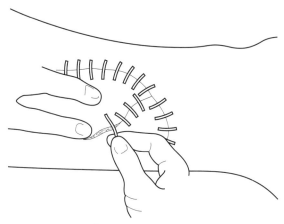

Fig. 11.16 Using Steri-strip® to close simple pre-tibial lacerations.

ⓘ **The limping child**

The limping child is a common presentation caused by a variety of pathologies. Accurate history and examination can be challenging in children of varying ages (Table 11.1).

Presentation
- Limp with hip/groin/knee pain
- Take a corroborative history from the parents; any history of trauma?
- The age of the child is paramount to directing the most likely diagnosis.
  - is the child unwell?
  - pyrexia of unknown origin;
  - irritability (especially in infants).

Examination
- **General:** temperature, pulse, respiratory rate.
- Developmental milestones and immunizations.
- Gait, leg length, range of motion.
- Look at the soles of the feet for signs of trauma, a very common cause of limp in younger children.

Management
- **Blood tests:** inflammatory markers are useful, although not diagnostic. Particularly high markers should prompt thought about septic arthritis.
- **X-ray:** although radiation exposure in children should be minimized, X-rays are helpful in ruling out potentially serious hip pathology. The X-ray depends on the condition, but an AP pelvis and frog-leg lateral are starting points. (see Fig. 11.17).
- **Ultrasound:** ultrasound is useful to detect effusions associated with a septic arthritis. If available at your hospital, discuss with a trained individual for a scan that day. Do not delay treatment for a scan.

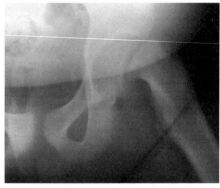

Fig. 11.17 Acute slip of the femoral epiphysis (SUFE).

Table 11.1 Differentiating paediatric hip conditions

Stage	Developmental dysplasia of the hip (DDH)	Septic arthritis	Transient synovitis	Perthes disease	Slipped upper femoral epiphysis (SUFE)
Typical age (years)	Neonates (screening); toddlers/adults if missed	<2	3–10	4–8	Males aged 14–26 Females aged 11–13
Sex predominance	Female	Equal	Male	Male (social class 4/5)	Male (obese)
Presentation	Screening; limp in toddlers	Systemic signs in infants, pain in toddlers, pyrexia and tachycardia	Acute painful limp, limited RoM	Limp, hip, or knee pain	Acute with painful limp, chronic with worsening limp
Pathology	Shallow acetabulum	Infection	No underlying abnormality	Osteochondrosis of femoral head	Slippage of femoral growth plate
Key investigation	Ultrasound neonates, AP pelvis X-ray infants and children	Aspiration Ultrasound if available	AP pelvis X-ray	Frog leg lateral pelvis X-ray	Frog leg lateral pelvis X-ray
Investigation shows	Abnormal hip anatomy	Urgent culture and sensitivity	Diagnosis of exclusion	Flattened and collapsed femoral head	Widened/slipped growth plates
Treatment	Control hip (surgical or non-surgical)	Aspiration, washout and antibiotics	Observe, NSAIDS	Observe, NSAIDS	Surgery to pin growth plates

Upper limb

☼ **Shoulder dislocation**

This section refers to acute traumatic dislocation of the glenohumeral joint, where >95% are anterior.

Presentation
- Anterior dislocation commonly follows a fall or other mechanism where there is forced external rotation in abduction.
- Posterior dislocations are associated with a seizure or electric shock.

Signs, symptoms, and clinical findings
- Pain and absence of active movement.
- Abnormal shoulder contour.
- Absence of sensation over the 'regimental patch' indicates axillary nerve compression/damage.
- Absence of hand pulses in a cold, pale hand suggests compression of the axillary artery and the need for urgent reduction.
- More extensive brachial plexus injuries can occur particularly in the elderly.

Investigations
- AP shoulder view and axial view show direction of dislocation (Fig. 12.1).
- Posterior dislocation gives a classic 'light-bulb sign' on AP – the glenoid head is abnormally oval shaped (Fig. 12.2).
- Repeat X-rays post-reduction.
- **Further investigation** (e.g. MRI): tearing away of the anterior capsule with disruption of the glenoid labrum results in a *Bankart lesion*. A *Hill-Sachs lesion* is a compression fracture to the posterior part of the humeral head against the anterior glenoid rim.

Management
- Reduction is attempted immediately in the ED. Assess neurovascular status prior to reduction.
- Spaso's traction technique is popular (see ▭ Shoulder dislocation, Reducing dislocated shoulders, p215).
- **Methods of analgesia/sedation**: include Entonox®, or commonly IV morphine and midazolam. Sedation should only be performed in the Resuscitation room with a trained nurse and a competent physician trained in advanced airway management, with full monitoring after written consent from the patient. **Do not use midazolam when on your own, and have an antidote ready (i.e. flumazenil).**
- Obtain post-reduction X-rays (AP).
- **Immobilize in a collar and cuff**: local policy may advocate other alternatives.
- Send to next Fracture Clinic for review and management planning.
- In patients wishing to continue to pursue sporting activities, acute repair is increasingly practiced.
- Early physiotherapy and mobilization is recommended in elderly patients.
- Weak sensation post-reduction may persist and can be re-assessed adequately at Fracture Clinic. Most nerve damage recovers with time and is initially treated with physiotherapy. Otherwise nerve conduction studies should be sought.

Associated fractures

- Fractures of the greater tuberosity normally reduce following reduction of the shoulder. They can be sent home and monitored in Fracture Clinic. ORIF may be required in due course for those with displacement.
- Displaced glenoid fractures will require CT after shoulder reduction, with subsequent ORIF for displaced fractures. If shoulder reduced, this can be done non-urgently.
- Fracture of the humeral shaft – closed reduction of the head first and monitor healing via Fracture Clinic. These require open reduction if this fails.
- Older patients may suffer rotator cuff tears.

Indications for acute surgical intervention

- Failure of closed reduction in ED necessitates MUA in theatre. Keep starved. If before midnight, place on the emergency list. If late at night (e.g. 04.00), place first on next available list.
- Failure of MUA in theatre requires open reduction (rare).
- Vascular compromise despite reduction; ischaemic limbs require a vascular surgeon's urgent opinion.

Who to send home and when to bring them back

- Once fully recovered from sedation, send home in collar and cuff.
- Keep in if not safe (e.g. elderly patient living alone; consider a rehabilitation bed, rather than acute trauma bed).

Pitfalls

- Not taking 2 X-ray views.
- Missing associated fractures.
- Missing posterior dislocations, especially those suffering from seizures with subsequent poor limb movements.

Rare dislocations

- *Luxatio erecta:* severe hyper-abduction leading to inferior glenohumeral dislocation; the arm is held over head. Vascular compromise, greater tuberosity fractures and rotator cuff tears are common. Reduction is with in-line reduction down the arm; GA may be needed if this fails.
- **Intra-thoracic fracture-dislocations** and **superior dislocations** are extremely rare. Call seniors for help early.

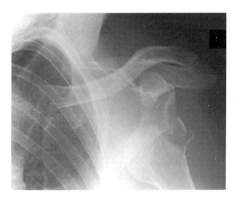

Fig. 12.1 Anteriorly dislocated humeral head now sits inferiorly and medially, underneath the glenoid rim and coracoid process. There is also a displaced fracture of the inferior glenoid, and so after reduction of the shoulder in the ED, the glenoid fragment required ORIF.

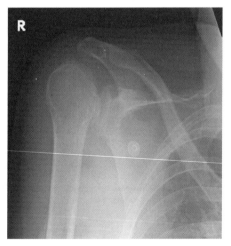

Fig. 12.2 Humeral head has an abnormal oval appearance. This is the *lightbulb* shape that suggests a posterior dislocation; clinical examination and an axial view are required.

Reducing dislocated shoulders

There are many techniques. These include:

Spaso's traction technique

Abduct the arm to 45° and apply in-line traction keeping the arm straight. Counter-traction is provided by someone standing at the head end of the bed and pulling a sheet wrapped around the patient's axilla (Fig. 12.3).

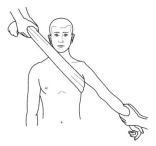

Fig. 12.3 Spaso's traction technique. Adapted from Bhangu & Keighley (2007). © Elsevier 2007.

Modified Kocher's

Not commonly used now. Flex the elbow to 90°, apply a little downward traction and slow external rotation of the shoulder. Pausing to allow muscle relaxation will allow the shoulder to spontaneously reduce. Finally, adduct the shoulder across the chest. If the hand on the affected side can reach the opposite shoulder comfortably, the shoulder is reduced. There is increased risk of fracture of the humerus if used in the elderly (Fig. 12.4).

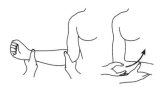

Fig. 12.4 Modified Kocher's technique. Adapted from Bhangu & Keighley (2007) © Elsevier 2007.

Reference

Bhangu A. and Keighley, M. (2007) *The Flesh and Bones of Surgery*. Oxford: Elsevier.

① Clavicle fracture

A fractured clavicle (Fig. 12.5) is one of the most common fractures and is most often treated conservatively. Complications are uncommon, but awareness of them is important as they are potentially serious.

Presentation

Fall directly onto the point of the clavicle, shoulder, or fall onto out-stretched hand (FOOSH, transmitted force from the hand).

Signs, symptoms, and clinical findings

- Pain, deformity, and occasionally bruising.
- The great vessels (especially the subclavian artery) can be damaged by bony fragments, resulting in an ischaemic limb.
- Neurological signs may indicate brachial plexus damage, which may accompany vascular damage.
- The skin over the fracture may be tented, putting it at risk and necessitating urgent reduction.
- High energy injuries may occasionally produce open fractures and are treated as such.
- A grossly displaced fracture with bone splinters can cause a pneumothorax (uncommon).

Investigations

- AP of the clavicle is usually sufficient – shows AC, sternoclavicular, and glenohumeral joints.
- Fracture is most common at the middle and outer thirds.
- The lateral segment is often displaced downwards.
- Imaging the opposite clavicle is useful only for detecting AC joint abnormalities.

Management

- >95% are treated conservatively (even if grossly displaced on X-ray).
- A broad arm sling supports the weight of the arm, which can help correct deformity.
- Immobilize for 2–3 weeks, although early active movements can be commenced, whilst still in the sling.
- Review in Fracture Clinic within 1 week for simple fractures.
- With this treatment, most will unite, leaving a bump underneath the skin. For the majority of people this is cosmetically acceptable.
- Tenting of the skin requires prompt intervention with ORIF.

Indications for acute surgical intervention

- Vascular damage/acute ischaemic limb needs urgent vascular opinion.
- Skin compromise.
- Open fractures.
- **Floating shoulder:** fracture of the clavicle accompanied by a fracture of the humeral shaft or glenoid.
- Soft tissue interposition between fragments leads to non-union; thus look for grossly separated bone ends.

Who to send home and when to bring them back
- Most go home with a sling, analgesia [e.g. co-codamol (paracetemol 1g QDS +/− opiate)], and review within a week in Fracture Clinic.
- Those with open fractures or vascular damage are admitted for urgent surgery.

Complications
- Vascular damage.
- Brachial plexus injury (uncommon).
- **Non-union:** affects around 1%. Internal fixation with bone graft are required for those with symptomatic non-union (e.g. young patients with pain).

Pitfalls
- Missing associated injuries, including those to the lung.
- Missing tenting of the skin.

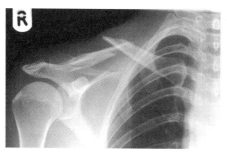

Fig. 12.5 Fractured clavicle.

ⓘ Acromioclavicular dislocation

Presentation
This most often follows a rolling fall onto the shoulder, with impact to the anterior shoulder.

Signs, symptoms, and clinical findings
Pain and deformity at the lateral end of the clavicle. With the patient facing you, the outer end of the clavicle on the affected side is more prominent than on the normal side.

Investigations
- An AP of the ACJ with the patient standing is taken. Bilateral views for comparison or weight-bearing views may indicate grade of injury (Fig. 12.6).
- The clavicle will be displaced by a diameter or more (of its own width).
- **Classification:**
  - *Grade I* – minimal separation (only acromioclavicular ligaments involved);
  - *Grade II* – obvious subluxation; still some bony contact;
  - *Grade III* – complete disruption, may benefit from surgical fixation.

Management
- A broad arm sling for ~3 weeks treats most (even those with gross instability).
- Those requiring high use from the limb (e.g. overhead manual workers) may benefit from ORIF.

Who to send home and when to bring them back
- Most go home with a broad arm sling.
- See again in Fracture Clinic within a week.

Pitfalls
- Missing sternoclavicular injuries.
- Missing injury by seeing a normal X-ray.

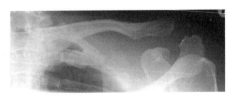

Fig. 12.6 ACJ disruption. The patient went home in a sling and was admitted via Fracture Clinic for open stabilization.

① **Sternoclavicular dislocation**

Presentation
- Fall or blow to the front of the shoulder (e.g. rugby-players).
- Occasionally spontaneous.

Signs, symptoms, and clinical findings
- Localized tenderness and asymmetry of the inner ends of the clavicle.
- Rarely, the inner end of the clavicle may come to sit behind the sternum, leading to signs of great vessel compromise and/or airway obstruction.

Investigations
- Request AP and oblique views of the sternoclavicular joint.
- Large disruptions may be visible; small one may not.

Management

Acute vascular problems or airway obstruction require urgent intervention. Both are usually relieved by manual reduction of the dislocation (lie supine with abducted arm, apply traction through the length of the arm).

- Gross displacements may require reduction under GA.
- A broad arm sling for 2–3 weeks treats most with a good result. Some residual deformity may persist and is acceptable.
- Continued instability may require open stabilization.
- Most go home with a broad arm sling; Fracture Clinic FU.

:⚙: Scapular fractures

Presentation
Direct blow, e.g. following a fall from a motorbike, producing pain to breathe because of the fractured scapular.

Signs, symptoms, and clinical findings
- Pain and decreased range of movement of the arm.
- Associated chest wall injuries indicate a high mechanism of injury and risk of intra-thoracic injuries, e.g. pneumothorax, haemothorax.

Investigations
- AP of the shoulder and trans-scapular Y views.
- A CXR is needed to exclude chest pathology.
- Look for fractures of the neck, spine, and coracoid process.
- Fractures of the glenoid require CT to assess the involvement of the articular surface.

Management
- Mostly conservative, with a sling for support and early mobilization as soon as pain allows.
- Early ORIF for glenoid fossa and scapular neck fractures may be beneficial.
- Most go home with a broad arm sling. Book into Fracture Clinic FU.

Pitfalls

- Failure to assess and identify associated underlying chest injuries, e.g. lung contusion. flail segment, pneumothorax.

- Failure to take note of the mechanism of injury.

ⓘ **Proximal humerus fractures**

Fractures in this region are common, especially in osteoporotic patients. Beware of interpreting complex fractures as simple fractures.

Presentation

- Fall onto outstretched hand or fall directly onto shoulder.
- Often occur in osteoporotic bone. High energy in the young.

Signs, symptoms, and clinical findings

- Pain, deformity, and swelling.
- Unable to move the shoulder.

Investigations

AP of the shoulder, with a second view (e.g. apical-oblique or translateral). Check for pathological lesions.

Classification

- **Start simple:** fractures are 2, 3, or 4 parts. 3 and 4 parts are likely to need ORIF.
- **Neers classification** describes groups I–VI:
  - *I* – fractures with minimal displacement (<1 cm) and minimal angulation (<45°);
  - *II* – anatomical neck displaced by >1cm;
  - *III* – surgical neck fractures displaced >1 cm or angulated > 45°;
  - *IV* – displaced fractures of the greater tuberosity (GT). Often part of a 3-part fracture (Fig. 12.7);
  - *V* – displaced fractures of the lesser tuberosity;
  - *VI* – fracture dislocations (typically fractured GT and dislocated humeral head).

Management

Management options depend on the type of fracture. However, many (especially those in the elderly) are treated with a collar and cuff where outcome is good. Specifics:

- **Non-displaced or minimally displaced** simple two part fractures with or without impaction (Group I). Treat with collar and cuff, and mobilize. Undisplaced simple fractures of the GT are treated in a collar and cuff for 2 weeks (watch until healed for late displacement).
- **Displaced anatomical neck fractures** (Group II): treat with a collar and cuff (reduce the head if necessary, as below). Fractures of the anatomical neck are at high risk of avascular necrosis; monitoring with delayed arthoplasty may be needed.
- **Severely displaced/angulated fractures** of the surgical neck (group III): many of these can still be treated in a collar cuff with a good result. However, for very severe displacement, closed manipulation may be required under anaesthesia; adduct the arm, push the shaft laterally and the head medially (bringing the fractures end together) and abduct the arm to close the fracture.

- **Displaced fractures of the greater and lesser tuberosity** (group IV): in isolation, some can be treated with closed reduction, although many require internal fixation. Since they are often part of 3 and 4 part fractures, ORIF with philos plate is used (control in a sling, CT scan via clinic, ORIF semi-electively by a shoulder surgeon). For older patients, conservative treatment with delayed hemi-arthoplasty can be used. In the fit elderly, immediate hemi-arthoplasty is an option. Best treated by upper limb surgeons.
- **Fracture dislocations:** simple two-part injuries (i.e. fractured GT and dislocated head) can be treated with closed reduction as for a dislocated shoulder. 3 and 4 part fracture dislocations are likely to need ORIF (e.g. with a philos plate) or even hemi-arthroplasty. The risk of avascular necrosis is high.

General management
- Provide early and adequate analgesia.
- Most treated in a collar and cuff, and brought to next Fracture Clinic.
- If a collar and cuff is inadequate, a hanging plaster cast will help provide traction.
- Those with obvious 4-part fractures likely to need ORIF can be admitted now, or discussed with and brought back to an upper limb surgeon's clinic.
- If sending home, consider social support in the elderly.

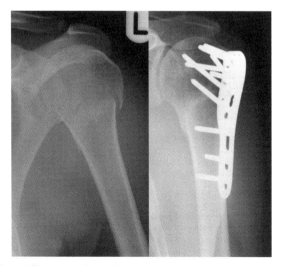

Fig. 12.7 This is a 3-part fracture (through the surgical neck and through the GT), which was treated with a philos plate.

⚠ **Humeral shaft fractures**

Fractures of the humeral shaft are common in adults, although uncommon in children. Complications include radial nerve damage and non-union. Fractures are considered and described as being of the proximal, middle, or distal thirds.

Presentation
- FOOSH or direct blow to the arm.
- Low energy injury may suggest pathological fracture.

Signs, symptoms, and clinical findings
- Pain, deformity, and swelling.
- Wrist drop and sensory loss over the first dorsal webspace in those with radial nerve damage (uncommon).

Investigations
- AP and lateral of the humerus. The shoulder and elbow should be included.
- Fracture pattern is variable; transverse, spiral, or comminuted.
- Look closely for pathological lesions.

Management

Simple fractures can be treated in a *hanging U-slab*, which helps reduce the fracture and maintain bony alignment until healing is commencing (2–3 weeks). This is then replaced with a functional brace.

- Displaced, comminuted, or angulated fractures may require ORIF in theatre. These should be treated in a simple U-slab and referred for specialist opinion.
- Those with radial nerve involvement should be assessed by upper limb surgeons. These may be treated conservatively, but may need ORIF if fracture pattern is unstable. If an open fracture, the nerve is explored.
- ORIF options include plate and screws, and intramedullary nails.

Who to send home and when to bring them back
- Patients are safe for home if comfortable in a U-slab, pain is well controlled and there is someone to look after them at home.
- Send to next Fracture Clinic FU.

Indications for acute surgical intervention
- Open fractures.
- Unacceptable position following PoP application. What is acceptable depends on age and functional requirements.
- Radial nerve palsy if develops post injury.
- Multiple injuries (especially to ipsilateral arm), bilateral fractures, two or more fractures in the same bone.
- **Pathological fractures:** after suitable work-up, an intramedullary nail can be used to treat fractures or for prophylaxis in suitable patients.

☼ Supracondylar fractures

Supracondylar fractures of the humerus are commonly seen in children and less frequently in adults (see Fig. 12.8). They are transverse fractures of the distal third of the humerus, just above the trochlea and capitulum. They must be assessed and addressed promptly to prevent serious complications. The classic deformity occurs when the lower fragment displaces backwards, and the sharp proximal fragment may compress the brachial artery and/or median nerve. Arterial compression is an orthopaedic emergency.

Presentation
- FOOSH in a child is the typical presentation, with pain and swelling.
- The child tends to hold the affected arm with the other.

Check for pulses and nerve function
- **Arteries:** presence and quality of the radial and ulnar arteries, as well as the brachial artery.
- **Sensation and motor function**: check all components of the median and radial nerve.

Absence or diminished findings suggests compression of the brachial artery, which leads to ischaemia; this is a surgical emergency. Failure to treat leads to irreversible ischaemia and subsequent permanent flexion of the fingers; this is a debilitating Volkmann's ischaemic contracture.

- Late signs of ischaemic compression include poor finger flexion and pain on passive flexion of the digits.
- Check for other injuries (including shoulder and wrist).

Investigations
AP and lateral of the elbow.

Management
- **For home:** if undisplaced, no significant swelling and pain is well controlled, discharge home with a backslab, analgesia, and Fracture Clinic FU. Undisplaced fractures can be treated for 3 weeks in a plaster followed by mobilization.
- **For theatre:** fractures with >50% displacement, >15% posterior angulation/rotation, or >10° medial or lateral angulation will require MUA in theatre. This is followed by plaster immobilization to beyond 90°. Obtain check X-rays in 2 plains.
- Unstable displaced fractures benefit from percutaneous wire fixation.

Managing acute arterial occlusion
- Remove tight bandages/dressings.
- Urgent MUA in theatre may restore pulses.
- Failure of pulses to return, but with good circulation (pink, capillary refill <3 s, good pulse oximetry readings) should be treated with 24–72 h of elevation and observation as most pulses return within 2–3 days.
- Failure to restore pulses and signs of ischaemia mandates surgical exploration of the brachial artery.

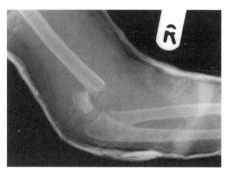

Fig. 12.8 Supracondylar fracture in a child. There was absence of a radial pulse, and so a backslab was applied and the child taken to theatre as an emergency. Under a general anaesthetic, the fracture was reduced with two percutaneous wires placed, and the pulse spontaneously restored.

Supracondylar fractures in adults

Supracondylar fractures in adults commonly have intra-articular extensions, often with a Y-shaped fracture configuration. All displaced fractures, except in the elderly, require open reduction and ORIF.

⭕ **Elbow dislocation**

Presentation

- Follows a fall, most commonly onto an outstretched hand, but also via a direct fall onto the elbow.
- Occurs in children and adults.

Signs, symptoms, and clinical findings

- Pain and absence of movements.
- Abnormal elbow contour. Loss of 'tripod' anatomy of the olecranon and epicondyles. The equilateral triangle formed by the epicondyles and the oleranon (as the apex) is distorted, whereas this is maintained in supracondylar fractures.
- Although uncommon, check for function of the ulnar and median nerves (motor function and sensation), and for distal pulses for brachial artery patency.

Investigations

- AP and lateral of the elbow shows the typical posterior dislocation of the ulna/radius relative to the humerus (Fig. 12.9).
- Associated injuries include epicondyle fractures and radial head fractures.

Management

- Reduction is carried out under sedation or GA.
- Slightly flex the elbow and pull steadily on the forearm, with gentle pressure on the back of the olecranon and countertraction from above.
- Recheck pulses and sensation. Place in an above elbow backslab at 90° and then obtain post-reduction X-rays; re-check for other fractures.
- Immobilize in an above elbow plaster case to 90° for 3 weeks.
- Home afterwards for Fracture Clinic care.
- If significant fractures or unable to reduce admit to Orthopaedics.

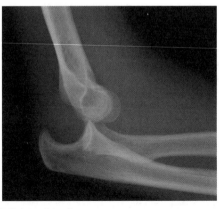

Fig. 12.9 Dislocation of the elbow joint.

:⚙: **Radial head dislocation**

Most radial head dislocations occur with an ulna fracture, thus becoming part of the *Monteggia fracture-dislocation*. True isolated radial head dislocation is uncommon, but important, and should be actively sought when looking at radiographs of painful elbows where no fracture is seen (especially in children).

Presentation
- Typically follows a FOOSH with forced pronation.
- Pain and decreased/absent movements.

Investigations
- AP and lateral of the elbow and *forearm*. Since isolated dislocations are rare, the forearm must be fully imaged to look for further fractures. (Note that bowing of the ulna in the presence of a radial head dislocation represents the greenstick component of a Monteggia fracture-dislocation).
- Look for a disrupted radiocapitellar line (Fig. 12.10). A line through the shaft of the radius should go through the centre of the capitelum no matter the position.

Management
Supinate the forearm with direct pressure over the radial head. Immobilize in a sling. Some require open reduction.

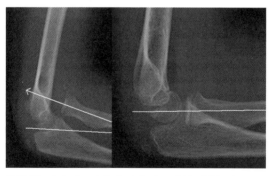

Fig. 12.10 Disrupted radiocapitellar line indicating radial head dislocation (left, arrowed) and re-alignment following reduction. Further X-rays should be taken to look for a second injury.

① Fractures of the olecranon

These are fairly common injuries, which often follow falls directly onto the point of the elbow. Good anatomical reduction is required for those producing intra-articular steps. Displacement of the proximal ulna fragment is common due to the attachment of triceps muscle – as it contracts, it pulls away the proximal olecranon fracture (Fig. 12.11).

Presentation

- Follows a direct blow to the point of the elbow or an avulsion injury following a fall.
- It is not an uncommon site of an open fracture in a high impact trauma.

Signs, symptoms, and clinical findings

Pain, swelling, and poor movements.

Investigations

- AP and lateral of the elbow shows crack fractures, displaced intra-articular 2-part fractures or communited intra-articular fractures.
- The proximal portion of the fracture displaces upwards due to the attachment and proximal pull of the triceps muscle.

Management

- Simple, undisplaced crack fractures can be treated in plaster for 3 weeks in children and <6 weeks in adults.
- Displaced intra-articular fractures require ORIF with tension band wiring, involving a tight figure-of-8 loop around short vertical wires (screws or plates can also be used). The fracture can be protected for a short while in an above-elbow backslab pre-operatively.
- For severely comminuted fractures, the olecranon can be excised and the triceps reattached to the remaining bone end. 3 weeks in plaster is subsequently needed, followed by physiotherapy. This also works for small, very displaced (by triceps pull) fractures of the proximal olecranon.

Who to send home and when to bring them back

If safe, these patients can wait at home and be kept on the rolling list. Send home in an above-elbow backslab in slight elbow flexion.

Investigations

Not realizing that this proximal ulna fracture is part of a Monteggia fracture-dislocation; look closely at the proximal radius for fracture and radial head for dislocation.

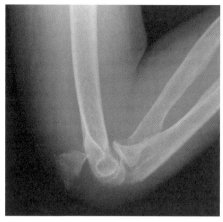

Fig. 12.11 Fracture of the olecranon caused by a direct blow onto the elbow. The proximal fragment has displaced due to the pull of the triceps attachment. This patient was admitted via the Fracture Clinic for ORIF.

⊙ **Other fractures around the elbow**

When involving the forearm bone, make sure to check for other fractures/dislocations (e.g. the 2nd part of a Monteggia injury).

Humeral condylar fractures

- These occur mostly in children.
- The lateral epicondyle is fractured much more commonly than the medial side.
- Small fractures on X-ray are, in fact, larger than expected, as the cartilage surfaces are not visible on X-ray, but give significant mass.
- Only small, non-displaced crack fractures can be treated in an above-elbow cast at 90° for 3 weeks.
- Complete fractures most often require ORIF as they are likely to displace with time. The consequences of displacement are significant, including non-union, early arthritis, and tardy ulnar nerve palsies (with medial condyle fractures).
- Admit from ED, and fix early or add to a suitable paediatric list.
- Manipulation followed by screw fixation is used.

Epicondyle fractures

- Occurring more commonly in children, following forcible abduction (avulsion of the ulna collateral ligaments).
- The medial epicondyle is more commonly affected, due to the common flexor attachment of the forearm muscles becoming avulsed during a fall.
- Treatment is largely conservative. Only major displacements and trapped medial epicondyles within the elbow (e.g. following associated dislocation) require ORIF.
- Ulnar nerve involvement can be treated with ulnar nerve transposition.

Capitellum fractures

- Occur following FOOSH, with force transmitted up the radius.
- Look for associated radial head fracture or dislocation.
- Treatment for small fractures is initially symptomatic with elevation, analgesia and support (e.g. broad arm sling). Most are suitable for home from ED with next Fracture Clinic appointment.
- Large fractures involve the articular surface and are displaced, often with an associated trochlea fracture. These require accurate surgical reduction. Backslab and admit from ED for elevation and upper limb surgeon review until ORIF.

Intercondylar fractures

Often forming Y- or T-shaped fractures due to force transmitted up the arm, these fractures may produce comminution. Non-displaced fractures can be treated in an above elbow cast, although many require ORIF (wires, plates, or primary arthroplasty) due to displacement.

Radial head fractures

Commonly follows fall onto wrist, where the radial head is pushed against the capitellum. Occasionally, follows direct trauma.

Signs, symptoms, and clinical findings

- Pain and swelling at the elbow.
- Pronation and supination may be maintained, although extension is limited.
- Holding the hand, and pronating and supinating the arm, whilst the thumb of the other hand applies pressure to the radial head causes pain.

Investigations

- Lateral and supination AP radiographs are usually diagnostic.
- Fractures may be hairline, complete non-displaced, displaced, or comminuted.

Management

- Simple, non-displaced fractures are treated with a collar and cuff for 2–3 weeks; then mobilized.
- Displaced 2-part fractures are treated with ORIF. Small fragment screws can be used.
- Severely comminuted fractures are best treated with complete radial head excision. Apply a backslab and book onto a suitable trauma list.

Radial head subluxation: pulled elbow

This typically involves a child being pulled by the arm in a longitudinal fashion, leading to the radial head being subluxed out of the annular ligament. The history is the key to the diagnosis. The child holds the arm with the elbow extended and refuses to use it.

Investigations

X-rays exclude fracture. The radiocapitellar line may be intact, although the arm will be maintained in pronation.

Management

- With the elbow in 90° of flexion, a thumb is placed at the radial head and the forearm gripped. The forearm is extended and then supinated fully, which 'screws' the radial head back into place.
- Check the child is using the arm normally again prior to discharge. Otherwise, consider an alternative diagnosis.
- No immobilization is required.

! **Monteggia fracture-dislocation**

This injury is a fracture of the proximal ulna with dislocation of the radial head (Fig. 12.12).

Fractures and dislocations of the radius and ulna are caused by falls or direct blows during defence (night stick injury).

Presentation
- Pain, swelling, and poor movements.
- Check and monitor for compartment syndrome.

Investigations
- AP and lateral of the entire forearm (elbow to wrist). Send back to X-ray if necessary.
- Look for forward displacement of the ulna fracture, with forward dislocation of the radial head.

Management
- Closed reduction can be initially attempted, although most require ORIF since closed reduction leaves inadequate results.
- Initially, place in an above elbow backslab with the elbow to 90° and elevate the limb on pillows.
- At surgery, the radial head relocates when the ulnar is fixed. Post-operative protection is in a plaster for 2 weeks then mobilization.
- Children may be treated with MUA and PoP.

Who to send home and when to bring them back
Patients should be admitted for monitoring of swelling, elevation, and consultant review in the morning. A CT scan may be needed for subsequent planning of ORIF.

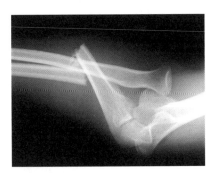

Fig. 12.12 Monteggia fracture-dislocation.

⊙ **Galeazzi fracture-dislocation**

This injury is a fracture of the shaft of the radius with dislocation of the inferior radio-ulnar joint (a mirror image of Monteggia; Fig. 12.13).

Management
- AP and lateral of the entire forearm.
- Admit and place in an above elbow backslab with the elbow to 90° and elevate the limb on pillows. Most require ORIF.
- Surgical fixation principles are as for a Monteggia fracture, but regular imaging is needed.

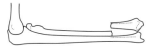

Fig. 12.13 Galeazzi fracture-dislocation. Adapted from Bhangu & Keighley (2007). © Elsevier 2007.

Isolated radius/ulnar shaft fractures
Single injuries to either bone can occur, but more commonly affect the ulnar. In children, they are mostly greenstick fractures.

Patients with a seemingly single forearm fracture or dislocation must be fully examined and radiologically investigated to seek a second forearm injury.

Management
- AP and lateral of the forearm.
- Closed reduction can be attempted, but most adults require ORIF. Transverse fractures are slightly more stable than spiral or oblique fractures, the latter of which are almost always unstable and require ORIF.
- The radius and ulnar are fixed with plates and screws through separate incisions. Plaster for support early post-operatively.
- Undisplaced isolated ulnar fractures due to direct blows are treated in plaster. Send home in a backslab.
- Isolated radius fractures are rare. Look for the second injury.

Reference
Bhangu A. and Keighley, M. (2007) *The Flesh and Bones of Surgery.* Oxford: Elsevier.

① Distal radius fractures

A Colles fracture, which occurs most commonly in osteoporotic bone, refers to dorsal displacement, radial displacement, and impaction occuring within 2.5 cm of the wrist joint. Dorsally-displaced distal radius fractures in young patients are different entities and are not termed Colles fractures. These are high energy injuries (e.g. motorcycle accident), they displace easily and heal badly.

Presentation
- **FOOSH:** forced dorsiflexion of the wrist; may be bilateral.
- In the young, these are high energy injuries.
- Check for other upper and lower limb injuries.

Signs, symptoms, and clinical findings
- Dinner fork deformity with pain on attempted wrist movement.
- Check for median nerve compression. Look for signs of new onset carpal tunnel syndrome.
- Occasionally, this fracture may be open, which requires management as such (📖 Open fractures, p146).
- Ensure you document hand dominance and occupation.

Investigations
- AP and lateral views of the wrist show typical findings (Fig. 12.14 – dorsal displacement, dorsal angulation, radial shortening, radial angulation, supination). There may be an associated ulna styloid fracture.
- Describe and document the degree of deformity.
- Check carefully for intra-articular components.

Management
The ideal aim is to achieve anatomical reduction:
- Closed manipulation for uncomplicated fractures is often attempted first in the elderly. Options include morphine and midazolam, haematoma blocks for the elderly, or Biers block.

Haematoma block

Clean the skin with an Alcowipe® or Betadine®. Wear sterile gloves. Palpate the fracture line gently using your fingers. Draw up 10 mL of 1% lidocaine into a syringe and, using a blue needle, insert into the area of the fracture line. Aspirate until the haematoma is drawn out. Now infuse the lidocaine, thus anaesthetizing the fracture.

- Contemporary practice is to fix all unstable Colles fractures irrespective of age; this commonly involves a volar locking plate. Admit for immediate fixation or add to rolling trauma list.

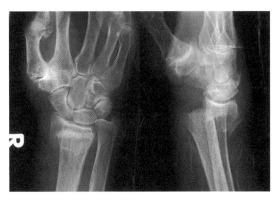

Fig. 12.14 AP and lateral X-ray of a Colles fracture showing dorsal displacement, dorsal angulation, radial shortening, radial displacement and supination of the hand. This fracture was manipulated to a better position, but still required ORIF with a volar locking plate.

Reducing a Colles fracture
- Take the patient to the plaster room. Aim to reverse the mechanism of injury; have someone pulling steadily on the forearm to provide countertraction.
- Dorsiflex further (to break the 'hinge'), then pull (to lengthen), flex the wrist (to correct the dorsal angulation/displacement), and then put into gentle ulna deviation (to reduce radial deviation).
- Alternatively, stand 'facing' the fracture, palpate the fracture line with your thumbs, and gently milk the fracture down into its normal position.
- Maintaining your grip, get someone to apply wool and then a backslab with crepe over it. Mould the plaster and manipulate further if needed to achieve a desirable position.
- Obtain a check X-ray. If the position is not satisfactory, someone more senior can try again and re-X-ray.

- If this is still unsatisfactory, consider admission for surgical fixation. If the deformity is minor and, taking into account the patient's age and occupation, it may be acceptable.
- Non-displaced Colles fractures in the elderly can be held in a backslab for 5–6 weeks. At week 1 the backslab is completed to a PoP, and serial check X-rays are used to check for slippage.
- Ulna styloid fractures that are displaced or angulated indicate disruption of the inferior radio-ulnar joint, and thus the need for manipulation of the fracture.

Indications for surgical intervention
- Open fractures.
- Displaced intra-articular fractures.
- Early reduction for early functional outcome, especially in young patients.
- Failure of closed reduction.
- Displacement in plaster cast (i.e. unstable fractures).

Who to send home and when to bring them back
- Most go home and can be seen in the Fracture Clinic the next day.
- Those likely to need surgery (e.g. young patients following high energy injuries) are either admitted from ED or sent home, and added to the rolling trauma list, having taken phone numbers and given instruction.
- The elderly with bilateral fractures may not be safe at home.

Complications
- Mal-union and stiffness.
- Late extensor pollicis longus tendon rupture (where it passes over Lister's tubercle) leads to poor thumb extension (flat palm on table, unable to lift thumb), and requires an open repair. Most often occurs week 3 to month 3.
- Carpal tunnel syndrome may be a late complication.

Pitfalls
- Missing the intra-articular component.
- Missing a scapho-lunate dissociation.
- Missing a late EPL rupture.

ⓘ **Other distal radial fractures**

Smith's fracture (Fig. 12.15)

- Fall onto the back of the hand with wrist flexed.
- 'Reversed' Colles – look for volar tilt.
- Apply the backslab to the volar aspect of the forearm.
- Most require ORIF due to instability. A buttress plate can be used.
- In severe displacement, initial closed MUA improves the position until definitive management.
- Book on to rolling list.

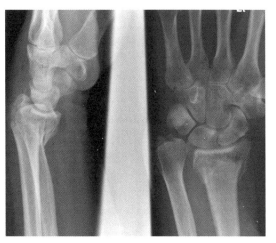

Fig. 12.15 Volar displacement of the distal radius indicates this is a Smith's fracture.

Barton's fracture

- A Barton's fracture is a volar distal radial fracture, which extends into the radiocarpal joint.
- Bring to next Fracture Clinic, book onto rolling list for a buttress plate.
- If the carpus subluxates forward with the volar component (which it often does), this can be reduced in the ED and then the patient admitted for definitive ORIF.

① Distal radial fractures in children

This is an extremely common fracture of childhood, where most occur following a fall and most are greenstick injuries (Fig. 12.16).

Presentation

- Most often a fall.
- Pain and dinner fork deformity are present.
- Check for median nerve compression. Look for signs of new onset carpal tunnel syndrome.
- Examine the elbow and fingers fully, as children may be reluctant to report other injuries.

Investigations

- AP and lateral views of the wrist.
- If in doubt, obtain full length forearm and elbow views to identify Monteggia/Galeazzi fracture-dislocations.
- Routine bloods are not required.
- Many are greenstick fractures, although 'off-ended' fractures occur (Fig. 12.17).

Management

- Non-displaced, non-angulated fractures are treated in a plaster cast for 3–4 weeks (backslab for first 2–3 days).
- Angulation in children can be accepted, as remodelling during growth will reduce the deformity. The angle accepted reduces with age. Typical limits are:
  - *aged <10* – <20° acceptable;
  - *aged 10–13* – 10–15° acceptable;
  - *aged >13* – <5° acceptable.
- Minor to moderate angulation can be manipulated as for a Colles fracture.
- Severe angulation and 'off-ended' fractures (marked deformity) require manipulation under anaesthesia. A periosteal hinge may need to be overcome and ORIF may be required depending on stability. K-wires or a flexible 'Nancy' nail (for more proximal fractures) may be needed.
- Following manipulation, an elbow backslab is applied with the elbow in 90° of flexion.

Who to send home and when to bring them back

- Careful discussion with parents is needed. Many young patients will remodel and so despite a few years of deformity, outcome is normal. Some parents will opt for MUA.
- For cases that require obvious or immediate MUA: admit.
- For borderline cases, most can go home in an above-elbow backslab. Tell the patients to starve overnight and discuss at the next morning's trauma meeting. If decided, the patient can come in immediately for theatre or if declined can be brought back to an appropriate Fracture Clinic.

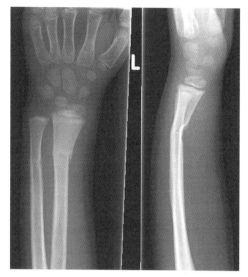

Fig. 12.16 AP and lateral of a greenstick distal radius fracture. The patient was admitted for an MUA and held in plaster.

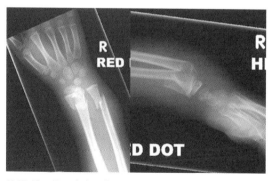

Fig. 12.17 AP and lateral of an off-ended distal radius fracture. This patient was placed in a backslab and admitted for MUA +/− ORIF on the next days' trauma list.

① Scaphoid fracture

The scaphoid is the most commonly fractured carpal bone, often occurring in young adults. It draws its blood supply from the radial artery, with 70–80% through the waist (middle), and 20–30% through the distal portion and waist (Fig. 12.18). There are two key concerns:
- Only around 70% of fractures are initially visible on X-ray.
- 5-10% undergo non-union, where the proximal pole loses its vascular supply and undergoes AVN.

Presentation
FOOSH.

Signs, symptoms, and clinical findings
- Tender scaphoid tubercle.
- Tender anatomical snuff box.
- Pain on telescoping of the thumb.
- Pain on deviation of the wrist over the scaphoid region.

Investigations
- **4-view scaphoid radiographs:** neutral PA, lateral, 45° supinated PA, and ulnar deviation PA (radiographers will do these). **You must ask for scaphoid views – not simply hand or wrist**
- 70% are identified on first radiograph. A further 20% are identified on X-ray at 10–14 days. Some may never be visible.
- Displaced fractures involve a step of >1 mm.
- Bone isotope scan or MRI from Fracture Clinic helps diagnose those not seen on X-ray. Early single slice MRI scan can give an early answer (e.g. student about to sit exams) – ask the radiologist if they can be fitted in.

Management
- **Severely displaced fractures** require immediate ORIF commonly with Herbert screws.
- **Non-displaced fractures** can be treated in a scaphoid cast for 8–10 weeks. X-ray at 8–10 weeks is required to check for non-union.
- **Non-visible fracture, but significant clinical suspicion**: put in a scaphoid cast and bring back to Fracture Clinic in 7–10 days. If still no fracture visible, but tender, refer for MRI scan for definitive diagnosis.

Complications
- **Subsequent non-union:** symptomatic disease can be treated with ORIF, using a Herbert screw +/– bone grafting (vascularized or non-vascularized). Asymptomatic disease can be treated non-operatively.
- **Osteoarthritis** is a well recognized late complication of this fracture.
- **Scaphoid tuberosity** fractures require only symptomatic treatment, with a crepe bandage or plaster for pain.

Scaphoid cast
Below elbow cast with slight wrist flexion and radial deviation, incorporating the thumb (Fig. 12.19).

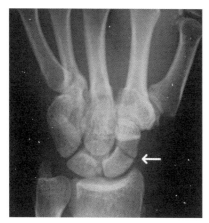

Fig. 12.18 Fracture through the waist of scaphoid.

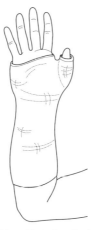

Fig. 12.19 Applying a scaphoid cast. Notice how the thumb is enclosed. Ask the patient to make an OK sign, then cast the bottom half of the thumb.

Indications for acute surgical intervention
- Displacement >1mm.
- Desire for early functional outcome in the young.

Who to send home and when to bring them back
- If safe to go home without driving, the patient can go home.
- If displaced and requiring ORIF, admit overnight if a theatre and suitable surgeon are available the next day.
- Otherwise book on rolling list if a senior decision has been made, or bring back to Fracture Clinic the next day for review and further planning.
- If a non-displaced fracture, send home in a scaphoid cast and bring back to Fracture Clinic in 10–14 days for further review and re-X-ray.
- If no fracture is seen, but still clinically suspicious, treat and bring back to Fracture Clinic for senior review.

Pitfalls
- Not taking 4 radiographical views to see non-obvious fractures.
- Initially, normal radiographs leading to a missed diagnosis.
- Seemingly minor pain causing a lack of clinical suspicion.
- Failure to monitor for non-union.

① **Other carpal injuries**

The lunate is the most commonly dislocated carpal bone. Other fractures and dislocations of the carpals are complex and hard to diagnose. Have a high index of suspicion (e.g. swelling and X-ray abnormalities) and refer early for orthopaedic opinion.

Lunate dislocation

The lunate is the most commonly dislocated carpal bone (the others dislocate relatively rarely). It most commonly occurs following FOOSH. (Fig. 12.20).

Signs, symptoms, and clinical findings
- Pain at the wrist.
- Signs of acute median nerve compression caused by the bone protruding into the carpal tunnel.

Management
GA is required, where manipulation or K-wire reduction are needed.

Other carpal injuries
- **Trans-scaphoid perilunate dislocation:** whole rows of carpals may be dislocated. Refer immediately to orthopaedics.
- **Fracture of the hook of hamate:** hamate views are needed. Treat in plaster and bring back to Fracture Clinic for further management.
- **Simple displaced and non-displaced fractures of the other bones:** these are usually the avulsion type injuries and are immobilized for 2 weeks only in a below-elbow backslab.

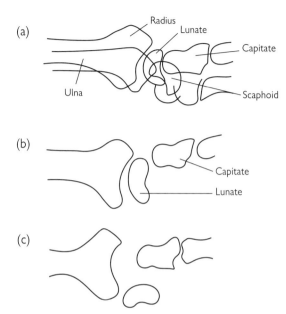

Fig. 12.20 (a) Normal lateral; (b) Perilunate dislocation; (c) Lunate dislocation. Reproduced from Wyatt *et al.* (2006) with permission from Oxford University Press.

Reference

Wyatt, J., *et al.* (2006) *Oxford Handbook of Emergency Medicine*, 3rd edn. Oxford: Oxford University Press.

⑦ Assessing the hand

Assessing hands fully is a skilful and detailed process. Describe the fingers as thumb, index, middle, ring, and small (1st, 2nd, etc, is confusing and don't say little as this can sound like middle on the phone). Describe directions as radial and ulnar (rather than lateral and medial), and ventral and dorsal (rather than anterior and posterior).

History

A detailed mechanism is vital:

- Establish hand dominance and occupation.
- Many are simple falls.
- For those with injuries from tools or equipment, find out details about the equipment, including whether tools were dirty or clean (e.g. old rusty blades versus a brand new circular saw).
- If the injury is from an animal, establish which animal, and whether it was a domestic pet or wild animal.
- For 'fight bites', establish how old the injury is. Note patients may be reluctant to give a true or full history.
- Establish if any antibiotics have already been taken.

Look and inspect

- Expose the whole upper limb on both sides.
- Look for swelling, deformity, skin breaks, abrasions, and other signs of trauma.
- **Fight bites** occur when a knuckle is pierced by a punch onto another individual's tooth. The tooth may pierce down to the joint. The finger moves afterwards, closing the puncture and a few days later infection develops. The joint is swollen, red and very tender. **These patients require immediate admission for antibiotics and drainage** (see 📖 Hand infections, p264).
- **Infections:** hot, red, tender, spreading cellulitis, generalized sepsis necrotizing fasciitis (this may occur from seemingly trivial injuries).
- Fractures and dislocations present with swelling and deformity.
- **Rotational deformities:** ask the patient to flex the fingers into the palm. The fingernails should all point in the same direction, towards the scaphoid. Rotation of a finger fracture causes rotation of the fingernail direction (Fig. 12.21).
- Assess and document skin loss.
- **Subungal haematomas:** heavy items dropped onto toes and fingers, or when they are trapped in doors results in haematoma formation underneath the nail. These are extremely painful. Drain with a sharp, sterile instrument, which is bored down through the nail (no local anaesthestic needed as the nail is insensate).

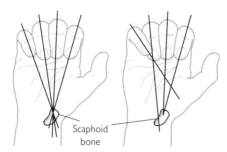

Fig. 12.21 Assessing for rotational deformities. With the fingers semi-flexed, all the fingernails should normally point towards the scaphoid. Adapted from American Academy of Family Physicians (2006). ©2006 American Academy of Family Physicians.

Feel

- Palpate for tenderness and temperature.
- **Sensation:** the radial border of the index finger and the ulnar border of the small finger are the most important sides for protecting the hand:
  - *median nerve* – test at the radial border of index finger. Covers the radial 3.5 digits;
  - *ulna nerve* – test at the ulnar border of small finger, covers the ulna 1.5 digits;
  - *radial nerve* – test over the first dorsal webspace;
  - for finger injuries (digital nerves), test sensation on the radial and ulnar side, including gross touch and two-point discrimination (e.g. with a paperclip).

Move

- Assess active and passive movements of all joints of the hand, and the wrist, elbow, and shoulder.
- Test motor function of the major nerves. Grip strength provides a gross assessment (Fig. 12.22):
  - *median nerve* – the OK sign tests the median nerve (ask the patient to make an OK sign with their thumb and index finger, and try to break the circle); also weak thumb abduction;
  - *ulnar nerve* – weak abduction of the small finger;
  - *radial nerve* – weak/absent wrist extension.

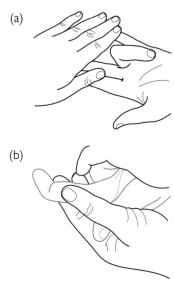

Fig. 12.22 (a) Testing the flexor tendons. Flexor digitorum superficialis (FDS). 'Try and bend your finger' (the examiner's fingers isolate movement to proximal interphalangeal joint); (b)Testing the flexor tendons. Flexor digitorum profundus. 'Try again to bend your finger' (distal IP joint is isolated).

Digital nerve blocks

- Use ~10 mL 1% lidocaine (**never** with adrenaline, as this may cause ischaemic necrosis of the distal appendage).
- Aim to infiltrate around the digital nerves in a ring fashion, so blocking all nervous supply to the digit (Fig. 12.23).
- Neurovascular bundles run alongside radial/ulnar sides of metacarpals and phalanges.
- Remember that the artery runs along with the nerve, so frequently aspirate to ensure you are not within the artery.
- *Remember to assess and document neurovascular status prior to ring block.*

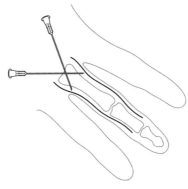

Fig. 12.23 Ring blocks.

Reference

Leggit, J. and Melco, C. (2006) Acute Finger Injuries: Part II. Fractures, Dislocations, and Thumb Injuries. *Am Fam Physician* **73:** 827–34, 839.

⑦ **Emergency referrals to a specialist hand unit**

Hand surgery is an evolving specialty, and high volume regional hand centres typically deal with hand emergencies on a 24-h basis. Both Orthopaedic and Plastic Surgeons run these units, although they deal with the same spectrum of injuries.

Who to refer to a hand unit

Different unit's policies will vary in whom to refer. Generally, those injuries which require referral to a hand unit are:

- **All flexor tendon ruptures:** these are complex injuries and require a high level of knowledge. Refer from ED.
- Extensor tendon ruptures distal to the MCPJs.
- Multiple tendon injuries.
- Thumb extensor tendon ruptures.
- Fractures distal to the MCPJs.
- Desire for early functional outcome in the young.
- Degloving injuries.
- Crush injuries.
- **Partial or complete amputations:** these are hand emergencies and should be sent urgently to regional units. Urgent ambulance transfer may be needed.

Transferring the patient

When referring to a hand unit, ensure you have complete documentation and X-rays to hand. Present the injury, mechanism, hand dominance, occupation, and treatment so far.

- Send copies of X-rays with the patient (hard copy or CD).
- The patient should be seen the same day. Instruct them how to get there, or arrange transport if unreliable or urgent.
- Dress any wounds in a moist skin dressing (e.g. paraffin gauze dressing (Jelonet®)), then gauze and a bandage. Do not place dry gauze onto wound as removing them can cause pain and further damage.
- Keep the patient NBM until seen by hand surgeons, and inform them why.

Hand patients requiring surgery to admit

Look at your local protocol. Typically includes:

- Open fractures.
- Hand infections.
- Complex wounds (e.g. tendon injury with fracture and soft tissue loss, such as major wrist laceration).
- Crush injuries/degloving injuries to the hand.
- High pressure injection injuries.
- Significant medical history.
- Unreliable patients (drunk, elderly, those living alone, those needing psychiatric care, etc.).
- Self-inflicted injury.

Hand patients requiring surgery to send home
- Simple laceration with suspected tendon or nerve injury.
- As above with a soft tissue defect <2 cm.
- Single closed fracture needing ORIF.
- Terminalization of fingertip.

☣ Digital amputations

These often occur in young patients at work and are emergencies. Hopefully the amputated part has arrived with the patient! Multiple amputations are possible.

- Remember ATLS principles. Seek other injuries.
- Digital/ring blocks are effective analgesia, but only use after assessing neurovascular status.
- Take a history before examining the hand.
- Treat as open fractures. Clean, photograph, dress, give antibiotics.
- These can be referred to hand surgeons via ED without delay (these can bypass orthopaedic teams).
- Keep the amputated digit clean and place in a sterile bag, and then in ice (not directly onto ice).
- If both neurovascular bundles to a digit are destroyed, there is major skin loss, or there is a significant crush injury, referral for completion of amputation may be required. Urgent assessment in microsurgical hand units is needed.
- For patients who have lost the amputated digit, completion of terminalization may be possible by local Trauma teams if expertise is available (e.g. by local hand surgeon the next day).
- These patients can often return home with adequate dressings, analgesia and oral antibiotics, to return to a suitable trauma list for terminalization (typically within 1–2 days).
- The age, occupation, hand dominance, and smoking status are vital in making these decisions.

Finger tip amputations

Finger tip amputations may affect soft tissues, bone, and/or nail beds. The difference between sharp and crush injuries is important, as is the involvement of the nail bed. Treatment depends on injury:

- **Affecting only soft tissue, no bone exposed:** primary closure with Steri-strip® for small injuries or suture for larger injuries (may need theatre).
- **Affecting soft tissue, bone exposed:** debride in theatre, primary skin closure, small flaps, or skin grafts. If inadequate skin coverage, the terminal phalanx may need to be shortened. This should not affect hand function.
- **Amputation through bone:** primary closure/grafts as above. If significant bone and skin loss, terminalization at the distal interphalangeal joint may be the best primary procedure.
- **Affecting only soft tissue, no bone exposed:** primary closure with sterile skin closure strips (e.g. Steri-strip®) for small injuries or suture for larger injuries (may need theatre).

Finger tip injection injuries

Injection injuries are caused by high pressure industrial pressure guns (e.g. paint, glue, oil, diesel, air), which penetrate the skin and inject foreign material under high pressure:

- The most commonly affected site is the finger tip of the non-dominant index finger. The patient is typically a young male.
- Although the penetrating injury is often small, the underlying injection of foreign material may be significant. The patient often presents with no or very mild symptoms and an insidious looking wound; you must remain highly suspicious of underlying damage.
- X-rays are taken and may reveal location of foreign matter or soft tissue emphysema.
- Injection injuries into the fingertips may enter the flexor sheath, which carries a poor prognosis, since fibrosis and/or infection cause poor function (especially with toxic material). Injuries into the palm have a better outcome.
- Direct injections into digital arteries may result in ischaemia.
- Ensure tetanus prophylaxis is up-to-date and start prophylactic broad spectrum antibiotics.

Patients should be admitted for emergency surgical debridement.

- Wounds are left open for serial debridement. Amputation may be necessary.

ⓘ **Tendon injuries to the hand**

The hand is a commonly injured structure and is injured through a wide variety of mechanisms. Patients are often young and require a high functional outcome, and so careful and thorough assessment is needed to identify all injuries.

Presentation

Mechanism and predisposing factors

- Often through traumatic injury with tools or instruments, although can follow FOOSH.
- Establish whether blades or saws were dirty or clean, and the likelihood of contamination (e.g. from metal shards).

Signs, symptoms, and clinical findings

- Pain and poor movements.
- Open wounds, where tendons are cut.
- Every tendon in the hand is assessed, as above. Specifically look for extensor tendon, FDS, and FDP function. The more complex hand/forearm muscles/tendons can be assessed if adequate knowledge, but often need full assessment by a hand specialist.
- Assess neurovascular status to each side of each finger carefully.
- Document accurately and clearly, which must include hand dominance, occupation, and tetanus status.

Investigations

X-rays of the relevant area are essential to rule out fractures (especially avulsion fractures) and foreign bodies.

Management

- Patients with tendon ruptures should undergo exploration and repair in an operating theatre (not in the ED).
- **Flexor tendon** repairs are referred to hand units, since surgical anatomy is complex.
- **Extensor tendon** repairs proximal to the MCPJs can be treated locally, by exploration in theatre by orthopaedic teams.
- Extensor tendon ruptures distal to the MCPJs should be referred to hand units since the anatomy is complex.
- EPL/EPB rupture to the thumb should be treated in hand units.
- Small wounds with contamination should undergo formal washout and debridement (not in the ED).
- If there is doubt about function (e.g. un-cooperative patients), formal exploration in theatre should be undertaken.
- Gamekeeper's thumb is an ulnar collateral injury (see 🕮 Injuries to the thumb, p263).

Who to send home and when to bring them back

The decision whether to admit or not will depend on local hand protocols (see 📖 Emergency referrals to a specialist hand unit, p252). If the
patient is to be sent home, they should have an appropriate dressing,
having had the wound cleaned, with antibiotics, and they are called in
usually by the hand co-ordinator.

⚠ Metacarpal and phalangeal fractures

Fractures of the hand metacarpals and fingers are common. Attention needs to be paid to the patient's age, hand dominance, occupation, as well as the position and displacement of the fracture.

Presentation

Mechanism and predisposing factors

- Falls, punches, direct blows, industrial accidents, crush injuries, degloving injuries (with/without fracture).
- Look for deformity, swelling, and rotation.
- Open fractures and open joint injuries are treated as such.

Investigations

AP and true lateral X-rays. In a true lateral, all the metacarpals are aligned.

Indications for surgical intervention

The following are generally unstable and require surgery:

- Spiral fractures.
- Multiple fractures.
- Severely displaced fractures (>10° angulation in AP view and >20° angulation in lateral view).
- Displaced intra-articular fractures.
- Fractures through the neck of a proximal phalanx.
- >50% loss of bony contact.

Phalangeal fractures

- **Proximal and middle phalangeal fractures:** when non-displaced, these should be treated with neighbour strapping. Displaced fractures are initially reduced and then assessed for surgery (see Fig. 12.24).
- **Distal phalangeal fracture:** most are treated with simple immobilization to begin with and then active use. Mallet finger is treated as such (see 📖 Metacarpal and phalangeal fractures, Mallet finger, p259).
- **Crush injuries** to the distal phalanges are often open and, if so, require meticulous washout in theatre. Terminalization may be the best option.
- **Dislocations:** confirm no fracture on X-ray, reduce with simple traction under Entonox® or ring block, and then neighbour strap. Send home with Fracture Clinic follow-up.

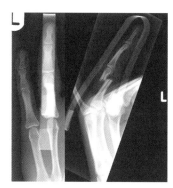

Fig. 12.24 This proximal phalanx fracture looks undisplaced on AP view. Lateral view reveals an off-ended fracture. This was reduced in ED under a ring block and neighbour strapped, although the patient was referred for K-wire fixation as the fracture was unstable.

Mallet finger

- A mallet finger is an avulsion of the extensor tendon from the dorsal aspect of the distal phalanx, quite commonly associated with a bony fragment.
- This is commonly managed in a mallet splint for 6 weeks, only to be removed for hygiene (when the finger is placed flat on a table and splint slipped out from underneath without losing full extension).
- In the presence of a large fragment, fixation should be considered. Bring back to Fracture Clinic.

Metacarpal fractures

- **Neck of the 5th metacarpal fracture:** these follow a direct blow to a clenched fist (e.g. punching; Fig. 12.25). Angulation >45° requires manipulation with local anaesthetic (LA) block (flex the MCP and push the finger up to correct the position of the distal metacarpal fragment. Some minor angulation does not affect function (Fig. 12.27). Rotational deformities and angulation >40–45° requires ORIF.
- **5th metacarpal shaft/head:** reduce if displaced and hold in a dorsal backslab. If unstable, will need ORIF (Fig. 12.26).
- **Middle and ring metacarpals:** stable due to surrounding structures. If undisplaced often treated with simple neighbour strapping of the corresponding fingers. Some may need a Colles cast (not too tight as these swell). Only if very displaced (i.e. off-ended) consider for MUA/ORIF.
- **Index metacarpal:** treat as for 5th metacarpal fractures.

Who to send home and when to bring them back

- Most can be send home in a backslab/dressing and managed via Fracture Clinic.
- For those needing surgery, attempt to correct major deformities under ring block, with simple traction, and neighbour strap or backslab.
- Only those with gross swelling should be admitted for elevation.

Plaster casts for hands

- In general, never splint the fingers in full extension, as flexion is rapidly lost. Cast with the fingers flexed as close to 90° at the MCPJ as possible.
- Leave uninjured fingers free.
- Advise elevation on pillows when at home or provide an elevating Bradford sling in hospital.

Pitfalls

- Applying plaster casts with the MCPs/fingers straight. They should be flexed at the MCPs.
- Not suspecting compartment syndrome with swollen, painful metacarpal fractures, especially after backslab application.

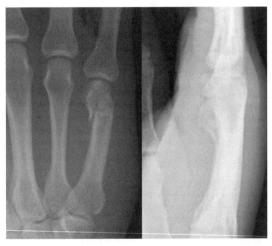

Fig. 12.25 This is a fracture through the neck of the 5th metacarpal caused by a closed fist injury. The displacement was minimal, so the fracture was reduced in ED with a ring block and a dorsal backslab (including the small finger) was applied. The patient was sent home and monitored in Fracture Clinic for displacement.

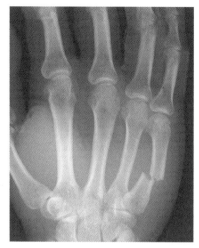

Fig. 12.26 Shaft of 5th metacarpal fracture with loss of bony contact and rotational deformity. The patient was admitted via the next day's Fracture Clinic and underwent K-wire stabilization.

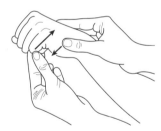

Fig. 12.27 Reduction of a neck of 5th metacarpal fracture.

⚠ **Injuries to the thumb**

Fractures, dislocations, and tendon injuries to the thumb are common injuries. Most can be treated in a plaster and brought back to Fracture Clinic, although appreciating unstable fractures which require ORIF is important.

Thumb fractures

Bennett's fracture-dislocation (Fig. 12.28)

- An oblique, intra-articular volar fracture to the base of the metacarpal of the thumb at the carpometacarpal joint.
- The distal metacarpal fragment displaces proximally.
- Minimally-displaced fractures can be reduced with longitudinal traction followed by pronation, and held in plaster cast or thumb spica.
- Larger fragments and unstable reductions require ORIF (e.g. percutaneous K-wires).

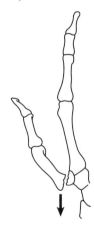

Fig. 12.28 Bennett's fracture of the thumb.

Rolando's fracture

- A Bennett's fracture that takes on the appearance of a Y or T pattern represents a comminuted 3-part fracture and is a Rolando's fractures.
- Marked comminution may be treated conservatively, large fragments require percutaneous fixation. Treat in a thumb spica and bring back to Fracture Clinic.

Other fractures and dislocations

- Other fractures to the base of the thumb (including greenstick fractures in children) follow similar lines. Closed reduction is used, with K-wires if this fails.
- **Dislocations to the thumb:** may be of carpometacarpal or the metcarpophalangeal variety. Attempt closed reduction by pulling in line to provide traction and hold in minor flexion in plaster. If this fails, ORIF is needed.

Gamekeeper's thumb

Forced thumb abduction may lead to rupture of the *ulna collateral ligament* (Gamekeeper's thumb). This is often the result of a fall onto an abducted thumb (Fig. 12.29).

- Test for instability by fully extending the thumb and stressing the ulnar side of the IP joint; look for mild to severe instability, and compare with the other side.
- X-ray may show avulsion fracture.
- Accurate assessment may still be difficult. In these cases and with high suspicion, apply a thumb spica, and bring back to Fracture Clinic.
- Marked ligamental instability or laxity are indications for surgery.
- **Associated avulsion fracture:** if present, small, non-displaced avulsion fractures can be treated in a scaphoid cast for 6 weeks (bring back to Fracture Clinic). Large, rotated, or displaced fractures are indications for ORIF.

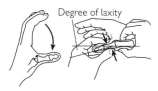

Fig. 12.29 Avulsion fracture associated with Gamekeeper's thumb and testing for ulna collateral weakness.

☼ Hand infections

Infections to the hand may produce devastating disability to often young, working patients if not treated early and correctly.

Presentation

Mechanism and predisposing factors

- Penetrating trauma is the most common mechanism.
- 'Fight bites' – human or animal bites.
- Beware predisposing factors, where small wounds can progress to serious infections (e.g. necrotizing fascitis) – diabetes mellitus, steroid use, immunosuppressants, intravenous drug abusers, HIV/AIDS.
- In the absence of penetrating trauma, haematogenous spread should be considered in its absence.

Signs, symptoms, and clinical findings

- Pain, swelling, and loss of movement.
- Tenderness, heat, erythema. Check/document temperature.
- Look for wounds and foreign bodies (e.g. a rose thorn, which the patient has not noticed).
- Patients may present having failed to seek earlier medical advice with significant problems, including florid sepsis, symptoms of bacteraemia, and necrotizing fasciitis.

Investigations

- AP and lateral X-rays to exclude fractures, foreign bodies, and seek out underlying osteomyelitis. Acute infections can occur with or without fracture.
- **Bloods:** inflammatory markers (WCC, CRP, ESR) are useful in monitoring progress.

Management

- Ensure **tetanus** is up to date.
- **Intravenous antibiotics:** for patients being admitted for antibiotics, first doses should be given before the patient leaves the ED. For those going to theatre, consider immediate antibiotics if there is likely to be a delay. Otherwise hold off so a fresh sample can be taken for culture during the operation. *Staphlococcus aureus* is a common causative pathogen; use antibiotics according to local protocols.
- Dress any wound, consider a loose backslab for comfort, elevate in a Bradford sling or high arm sling.
- If for referral to a hand unit, kept NBM and arrange transfer to a hand unit.

Fight bites

- These are penetrating injuries to a closed fist, often when the knuckle makes contact with someone else's teeth. Infection sets in a few days later. Worried patients may deny the mechanism but appearances are typical.
- The knuckle is hot, swollen, and tender.

Patients with fight bites should be admitted for surgical washout of the joint with copious irrigation. Admit, X-ray, elevate, give IV antibiotics, prepare for theatre.

Pyogenic flexor tenosynovitis

- This is infection within the flexor sheath and is an orthopaedic emergency. Penetrating trauma is usually responsible.
- Pathogens multiply rapidly within this closed space.
- Left untreated, inflammation leads to loss of the gliding surfaces of the sheath, with subsequent scarring, adhesions, and permanent debilitating flexion of the digits. There are 4 classic signs:
  - fingers held in slight flexion;
  - swelling;
  - tenderness along the flexor sheath;
  - pain with passive extension of the fingers.
- Beware that these may be absent in those with recent antibiotic treatment, immunocompromised state, or very early infection.
- **Early surgical debridement and antibiotics are the mainstay of treatment.** Thorough and copious washout of the flexor sheath is needed, cultures sent, and empiric antibiotics started.
- These are best dealt with in a hand unit. Keep starved, immobilize for analgesia, elevate the arm, consider antibiotics in the ED after liaison with hand units (especially if there is likely to be any delay to theatre).

Paronychia

- Infection of the epidermis (nail-fold) surrounding the fingernail.
- If early (little cellulitis, no fluctuance) consider oral antibiotics.
- If pus/abscess is present, surgical incision, and drainage under digital nerve block is needed.

Felon: pulp infections

- A felon is an abscess of the distal finger pulp.
- Penetrating trauma is the normal cause, such as thorns, nails, or broken blisters.
- X-rays should be taken to assess for osteomyeltitis.
- Early infection may respond to elevation and antibiotics.
- Established infection requires incision and drainage.

Pitfalls

Under-estimating severity, especially when dealing with pyogenic flexor tenosynovitis.

Spine

☼ Spinal fractures

Fractures through the spine should be considered by anatomical regions – cervical, thoracic, and lumbar. Remember with one spinal fracture following trauma (e.g. thoracic), there is a 10–20% chance of a second fracture elsewhere in the spine – actively seek it and keep the whole spine immobilized until excluded.

Cervical fractures and dislocations

- **Flexion-rotation injuries:** these may be stable or unstable, and may produce fractures and/or dislocations. Injuries include anterior wedge fractures, unilateral and bilateral facet joint dislocation, avulsion of spinous processes.
- **Facet joint dislocations** are major and unstable injuries, with either impending or established spinal cord injury. Immobilize fully and minimize movement. Organize urgent CT scan. A halo brace may be needed following reduction, or surgical reduction and stabilization is required (Fig. 13.1). Seek senior help early; discussion with spinal surgeons will be needed.

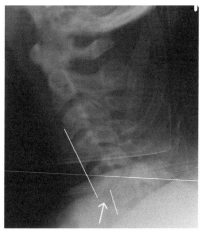

Fig. 13.1 The white line indicates disruption of the anterior spinal line. The C5 vertebrae is displaced by 50% compared with C6, indicating bifacet dislocation. The film is inadequate, but guided the need for careful handling and immediate CT of the whole spine.

- **C1 (Jefferson) fracture:** the classic fracture pattern is quadripartite fracture, where there is axial loading and thus a 'burst' fracture. Obtain urgent CT scan and spinal surgeon opinion. Immobilize with halo brace. Gross disruption of the ring may be unstable and cause immediate death.

- **Odontoid peg fractures:** the peg may be fractured, or may become unstable when its restraining transverse ligament is disrupted (treat with immobilization and urgent traction). There are 3 types of peg fracture:
  - *type I* – tip of the peg; stable, rare, good prognosis, treat with collar;
  - *type II* – junction of head and body; most common, unstable;
  - *type III* – below the junction; unstable.
- **Hangman's fractures:** a hyperextension injury with fracture of pedicles of C2. There may be disruption of C2–C3 junction. Immobilize, call seniors early on, arrange CT scan, discuss with spinal surgeons. Options include skull traction for 6 weeks or surgical fixation (correct terminology is the 'Hanged Man's' fracture).
- **C3 to C7 fractures:** may be stable or unstable depending on the fracture configuration. Immobilize, obtain CT, and discuss with spinal surgeons.

Thoracic/lumbar spine fractures

- Many are *wedge fractures* following falls. Most are stable fractures (*anterior column only*) are treated with bed rest and analgesia until the acute pain resolves, followed by gradual and controlled mobilization.
- Patients with fractures involving *two or three columns* (e.g. burst fractures, dislocations) should be immobilized on a spinal bed and spinal surgeon advice sought.
- **Chance fracture:** caused by violent forward flexion, these injuries may involve bone, ligament and/or disc, and mostly occur at the thoraco-lumbar junction (T12–L2). Typically, occurring after the restraint from a head-on impact whilst wearing a lap belt, they are associated with intra-abdominal injuries. Pure ligamentous injuries may not show bony injury; the bony ones will have loss of the 'owl's eye' sign. The anterior, middle, and posterior columns fail under tension. Fractures may be treated operatively or non-operatively, based on pattern/stability (consider CT).
- In older patients consider pathological fractures.
- Fractures of the sacrum and coccyx are considered to be part of a pelvic fracture (see 📖 Types of pelvic fractures, Sacral fractures, p169; 📖 Types of pelvic fractures, Coccyx fractures, p169).

Pitfalls

- **Fractures at the thoraco-lumbar junction are commonly missed** due to the failure to appreciate the mechanism of injury (e.g. ejection from car), major distracting injury, or concentrating on the cervical spine.
- Not seeking for or appreciating a second fracture/dislocation; the whole spine must be considered.

⚙️ Spinal cord compression and cauda equina syndrome

Acute compression of the spinal cord is an orthopaedic emergency. Compression above L1/2 affects the spinal cord and below that affects the nerves of the cauda equina. Presentation may be at impending, early, or late stages of compression.

Pathology
- **Prolapsed intervertebral disc:** prolapse of a disc may compress the spinal cord/cauda equina if it is an acute, large central disc prolapse (Fig. 13.2). Small lateral prolapses may compress the spinal nerve roots, giving rise to much less severe symptoms (= sciatica, not an emergency).
- **Trauma:** fractures of the vertebrae producing retropulsed bone into the spinal canal, foreign bodies, expanding haematomas.
- **Tumour:** secondary tumours are much more common than primaries (e.g. lumbar spine deposits from prostate cancer).
- **Infection:** e.g. spinal abscess.

Presentation
Presentation is typically with the triad of pain, lower limb sensory changes, and sphincter disturbance.
- **Pain:** it is important to differentiate between 'simple' sciatica pain and more serious pathology. Compression typically causes severe, constant pain *below the knees*. Straight leg raise exacerbates the pain.
- **Sensory disturbance:** test and map the dermatomal distribution of sensation changes carefully, as this helps identify the spinal level affected.
- **Sphincter disturbance:** S2–4 spinal segments give rise to the pudendal nerve, supplying sensation and motor function to the bowels and bladder. Those affected typically cannot feel the passage of motion, may be constipated, and have altered urinary function (e.g. sudden incontinence or painless retention). Patients in pain who lie in bed may go into physiological urinary retention, but they maintain peri-anal tone and sensation.

Power can be affected by pain and may be misleading if considered alone. However, in the presence of this triad, power is often pathologically affected and so try to delineate the affected myotomes.

Red flag symptoms of spinal cord compression
Consider with new onset bilateral pain below the knees, dermatomal sensory loss and/or bladder and bowel dysfunction.

Investigations
- **Bloods:** inflammatory markers are useful to exclude infection.
- **X-rays:** of the lumbar spine may show degenerative changes or acute changes (e.g. spondyliothesis).
- **MRI** is the definitive test.

Management
- Catheterize to protect the bladder (especially if distended and non-tender).
- Obtain MRI and discuss with specialist centres. For non-traumatic acute compression, decompression within 6 hours is the definitive treatment.
- Radiotherapy can be used in conjunction with specialists, particularly if palliative.
- There is no current indications for steroids.

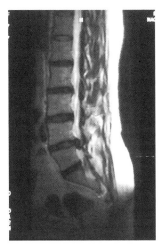

Fig. 13.2 MRI showing L4/5 intervertebral disc prolapse causing compression of the cauda equina.

Dealing with 'simple' back pain
Common causes of simple back pain include simple sciatica and mechanical back pain.
- **Exclude spinal cord compression:** take full history and examination. Ensure **YOU** do the PR (do not rely on prior examination).
- **Features of simple sciatica:** include pain below the knee, radicular pain or numbness, dermatomal sensory changes, and myotonal weakness; no bowel or bladder symptoms.
- In the absence of red flag signs, most acute back settles in 6 weeks with analgesia and active mobilization.
- Treat with analgesia and diazepam; mobilize with physiotherapists in ED or GP.
- Discharge if mobile. Otherwise admission for analgesia and in-patient physiotherapy is required. Discharge to the GP for follow-up providing there is good home support and good pain control.
- Progressive neurology is an indication for urgent MRI and spinal surgeon opinion.

☼ Spinal cord injuries

With or without fractures, the spinal cord can be damaged. Injuries without fracture may occur due to vascular insults or extension/flexion injuries. Complete spinal cord transection leads to complete loss of all function below that level. Otherwise, incomplete cord injuries may occur, which have very variable patterns. Knowledge of the location of ascending and descending pathways is needed to assess fully. Treat as for any spinal injury with initial immobilization and subsequent urgent CT/MRI.

Summary of functions of spinal pathways

- **Spinothalamic tract:** an ascending sensory pathway conveying pain and temperature. Cross over at the level of entry into the spinal cord.
- **Dorsal tracts:** an ascending sensory pathway conveying fine touch and proprioception/vibration. Cross over in the medulla.
- **Corticospinal tracts:** a descending motor pathway conveying motor function. Cross over in the pyramids of the medulla.

Spinal cord transection

- **Complete spinal cord transection:** leads to a complete loss of function below the level of injury. No further recovery occurs.
- **Incomplete spinal cord transections:** there is a variable pattern of distal function. Recovery and residual function varies according to the pattern and severity of injury.

Anterior cord syndrome

- May be caused by flexion injuries or venous thrombosis.
- Damage to the corticospinal tracts and spinothalamic tracts; sparing of the dorsal columns. This gives rise to a loss of motor function and pain/temperature, with preservation of proprioception.

Central cord syndrome

Typically affecting the elderly with degenerative bony changes. Variable levels of quadriplegia with arms affected more than legs (upper limb motor fibres placed more centrally). Sensory involvement is variable.

Posterior cord syndrome

Affecting the dorsal columns, leading to a loss of fine touch/proprioception, but preservation of motor function.

Brown-Sequard syndrome

- A hemisection of the spinal cord (e.g. following penetrating injury.
- There is *ipsilateral* loss of motor function and proprioception, and *contalateral* loss of pain/temperature.
- Treat with immobilization, urgent imaging, and advice from spinal unit.

SCIWORA – spinal cord injury without radiological abnormality

- This typically occurs in young children, <8 years old, but can also be present in adults.
- The increased flexibility in paediatric spines can allow severe spinal injury to occur in the absence of abnormal X-ray findings.
- There is a history of, or examination findings of, neurological deficit.
- Immobilization and arrange urgent MRI scan. Senior opinion is needed to direct further management.

Spinal shock

- Spinal shock is a loss of sensation, motor function, and reflexes following spinal cord injury, which is followed by a gradual recovery of reflexes below the level of injury.
- It typically lasts 24–48 h, and return of reflexes signals the end of spinal shock. The *bulbocavernosus reflex* is one of the first reflexes to return. Hyperflexia and hypertonia occur following resolution.
- Return of sensory and motor function may accompany return of reflexes, and indicates incomplete spinal injury.
- However, absence of motor and sensory function, despite return of reflexes (in particular the bulbocavernosus reflex), indicates complete spinal cord injury and prognosis is poor.

Index

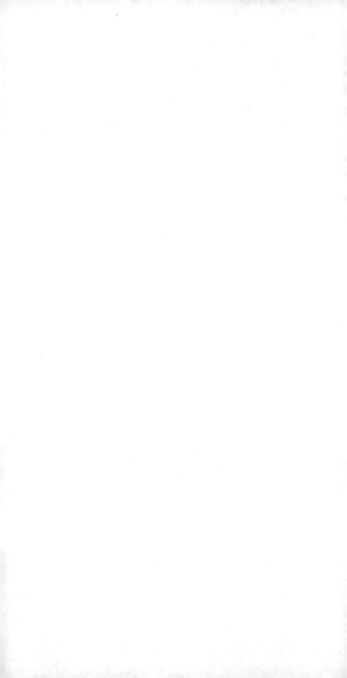